BEN & OWEN FRANKS
TRAINING TOUGH

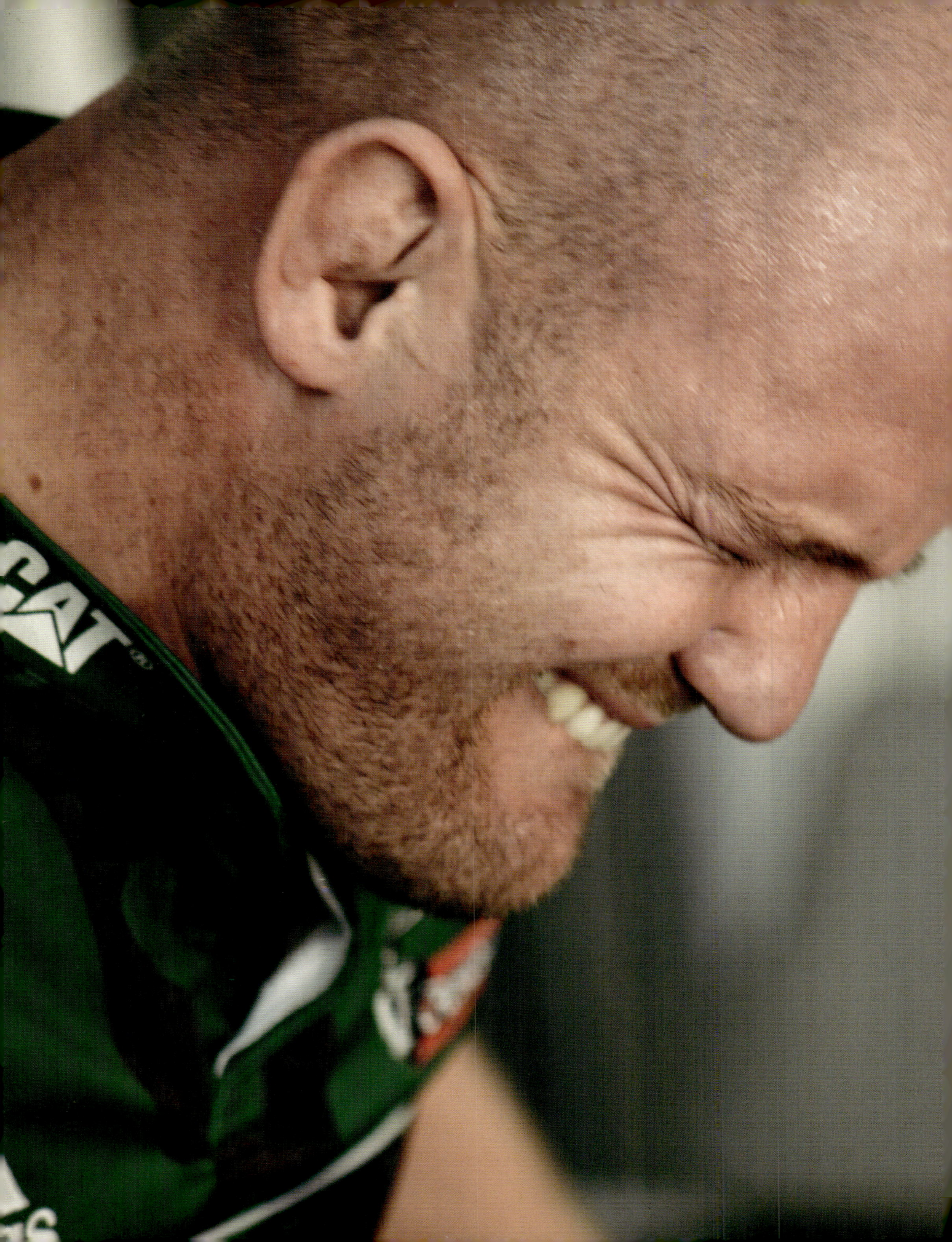

BEN & OWEN FRANKS
TRAINING TOUGH
WORKING OUT WITH THE FRANKS BROTHERS

With James McLeod

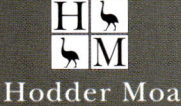

Hodder Moa

Photo credits
James McLeod: 2–3, 5, 6–7, 8 (centre), 10, 13, 14–15, 17, 18–19, 30, 32–33, 34, 35, 36, 38–39, 40, 41, 42, 43, 44, 45, 46, 47, 48, 49, 50, 51, 53, 54, 55, 56, 57, 58, 59, 60, 61, 62, 63, 64, 65, 66–67, 68, 69, 70, 71, 72, 73, 74, 75, 76, 77, 78, 79, 80, 81, 83, 84–85, 86, 87, 88, 89, 90, 91, 92, 93, 94, 95, 96, 97, 98, 99, 100, 101, 102, 103, 104, 105, 106–107, 108, 109, 110, 111, 112, 113, 114–115, 116, 117, 118, 119, 120, 121, 122, 123, 124, 125, 126, 127, 128, 129, 130, 131, 132, 133, 137, 140.
Getty: 8 (top and bottom), 22–23, 24, 25, 26 (top and bottom), 27, 28, 52 (top and bottom).
Franks family: 11 (top and bottom), 12, 16, 21.

National Library of New Zealand Cataloguing-in-Publication Data

Franks, Ben, 1984-
Training tough / Ben & Owen Franks with James McLeod.
ISBN 978-1-86971-277-8
1. Franks, Ben, 1984- 2. Franks, Owen, 1987- 3. Rugby football
—Training—New Zealand. 4. Rugby Union football—Psychological aspects. I. Franks, Owen, 1987- II. McLeod, James.
III. Title.
796.333092293—dc 23

A Hodder Moa Book
Published in 2013 by Hachette New Zealand Ltd
4 Whetu Place, Mairangi Bay
Auckland, New Zealand
www.hachette.co.nz

Designed and produced by Hachette New Zealand Ltd
Printed by Everbest Printing Co. Ltd., China

To Mum and Nana

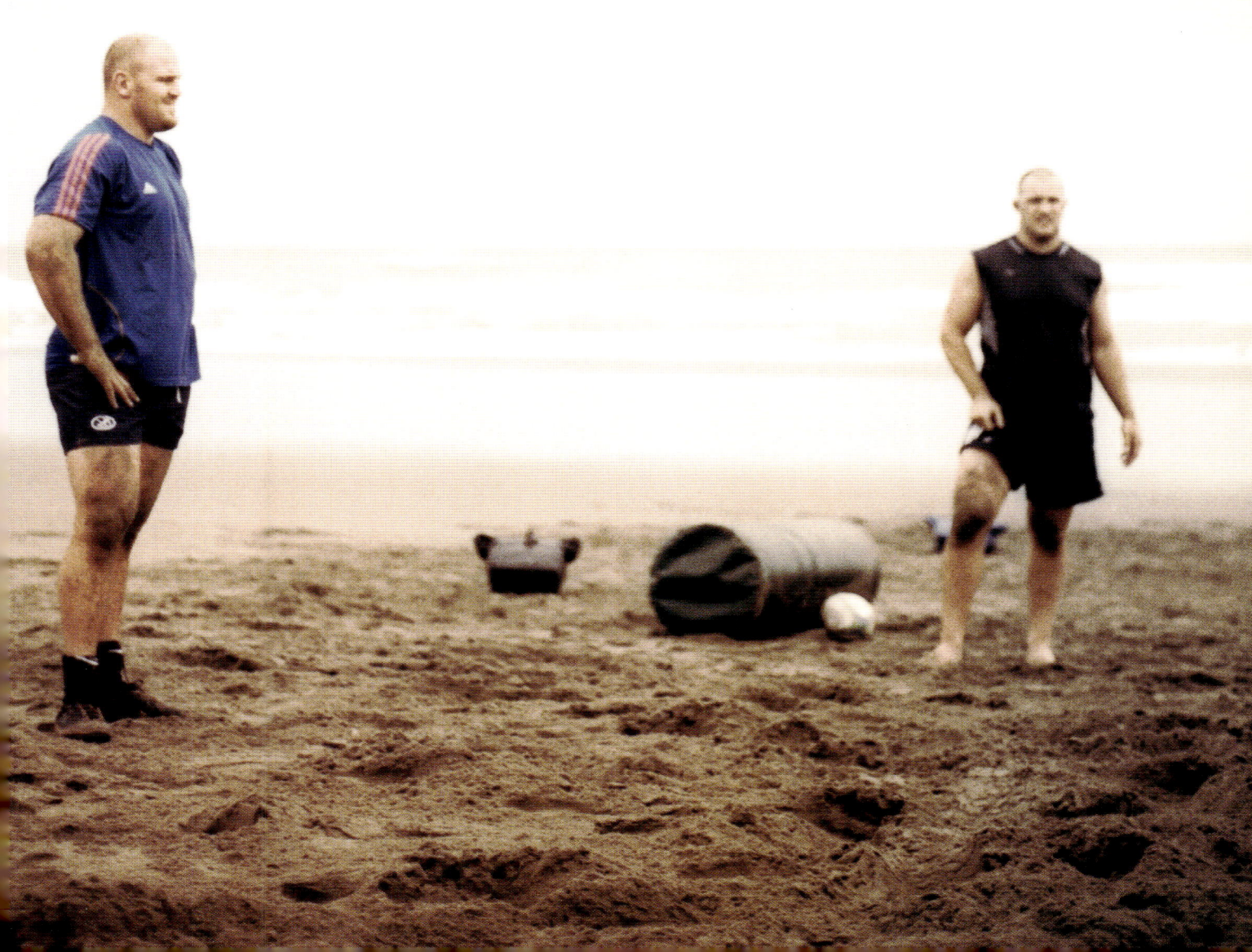

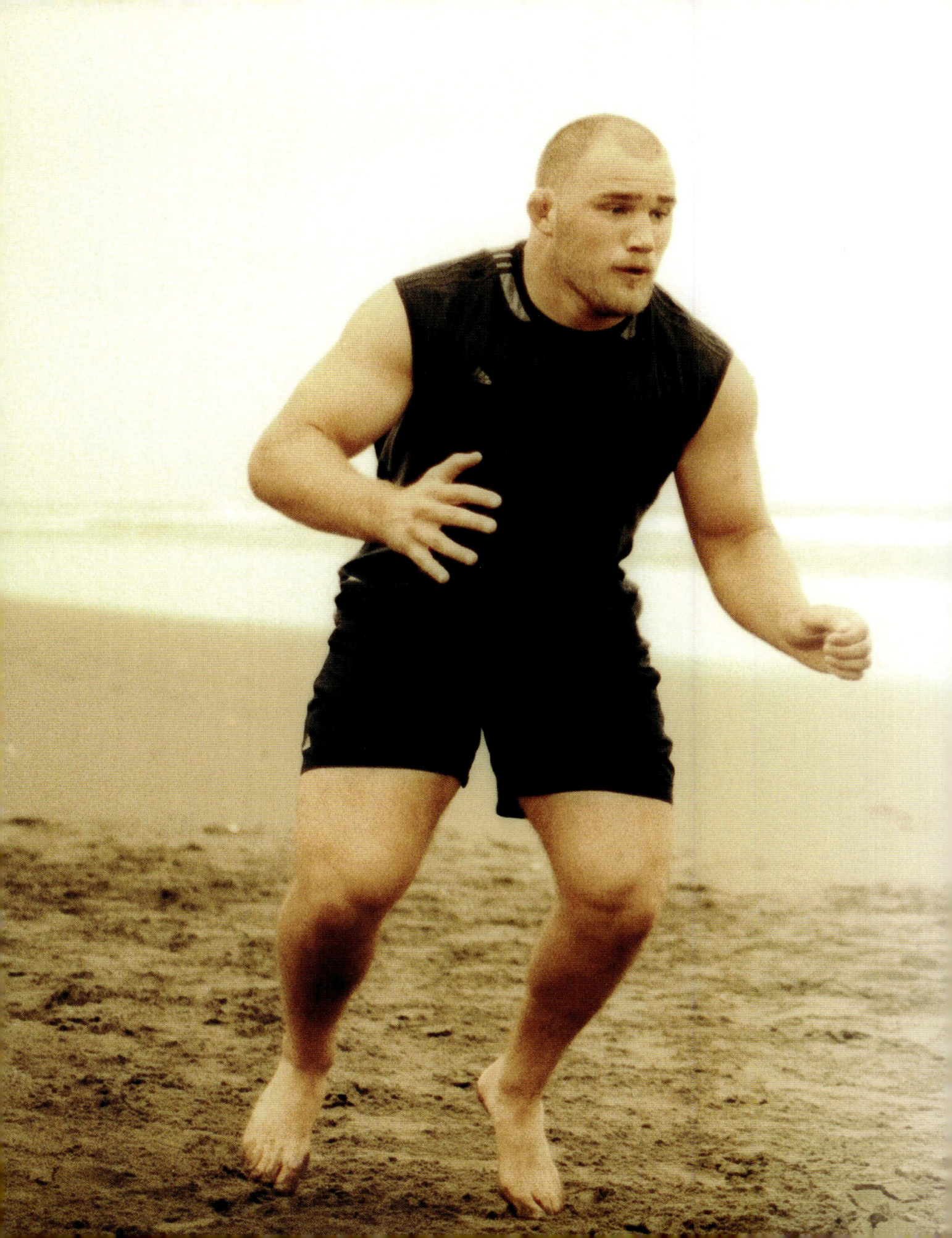

Contents

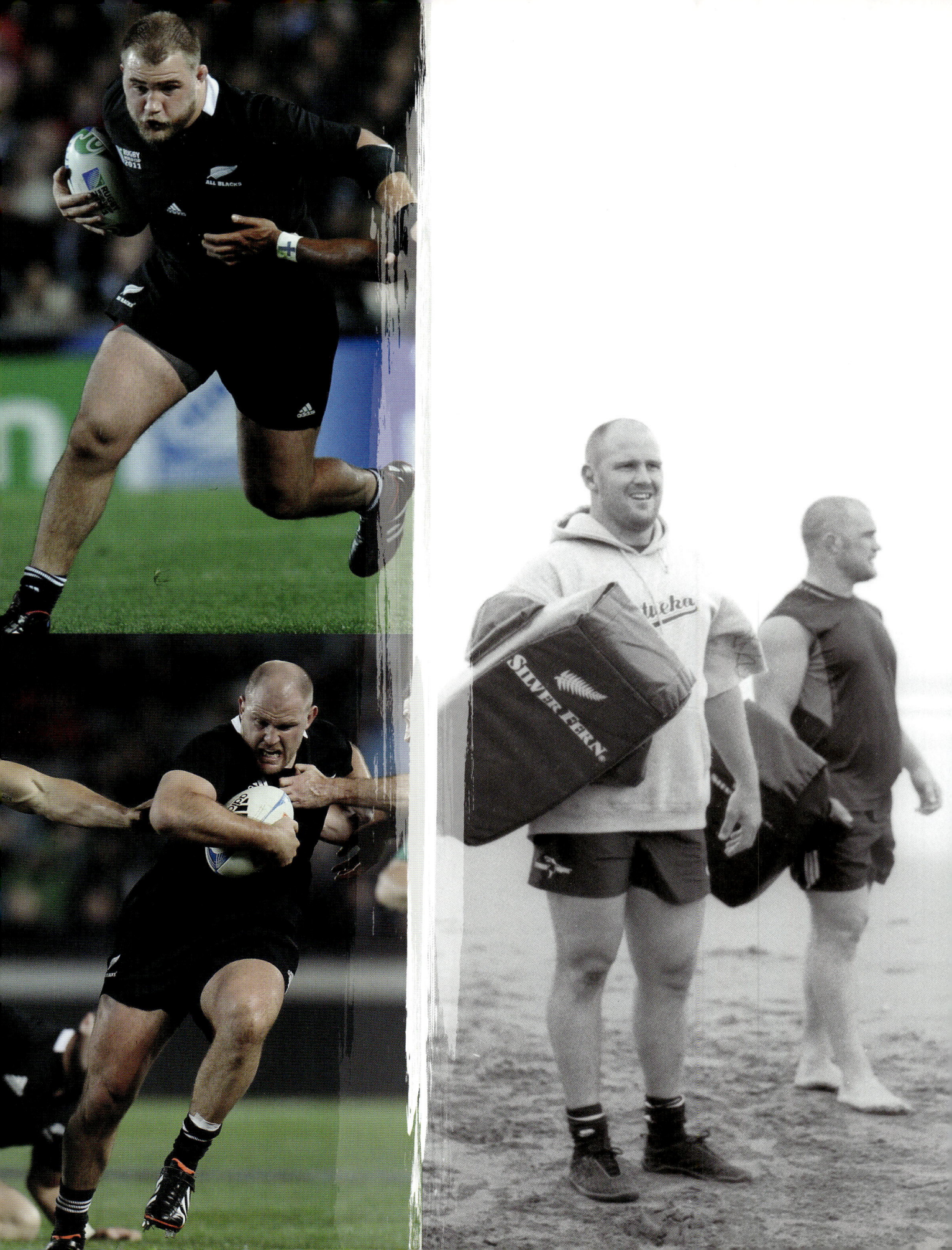

TO BE FRANKS

By Phil Gifford

To the New Zealand rugby public Owen and Ben Franks are a terrific reminder of another era, when All Black tight forwards looked like they'd driven to the game in a ute fresh from shearing 500 sheep, or stalking deer in rugged back country.

They're the embodiment of the attitude the legendary Kevin Skinner, the man who tamed the South African front row in 1956, brought to the field, an approach he summed up by saying, 'When you wear the All Black jersey you must bend the knee to no man.'

To Crusaders' coach Todd Blackadder Ben and Owen are 'probably the most professional rugby players I've ever come across. Just their preparation, their planning, their nutrition, their work ethic, they leave no stone unturned. They're extremely dedicated to their profession, and they've got a bit of a bloody cold steel edge to them.'

Former All Blacks prop, and Crusaders' scrum coach, Dave Hewett told a journalist the Franks brothers are a hybrid of old and new. 'They're uncompromising and won't back down from anything, but they're not dirty at all. They're consummate professionals. They love their scrummaging, and that's where they measure themselves. They love that confrontational aspect. Their habits around recovery and training are great. Their nutritional adherence is also phenomenal.

Far left: Owen (top) and Ben carrying strongly for the All Blacks.
Centre: Ben and Owen training on the beach.

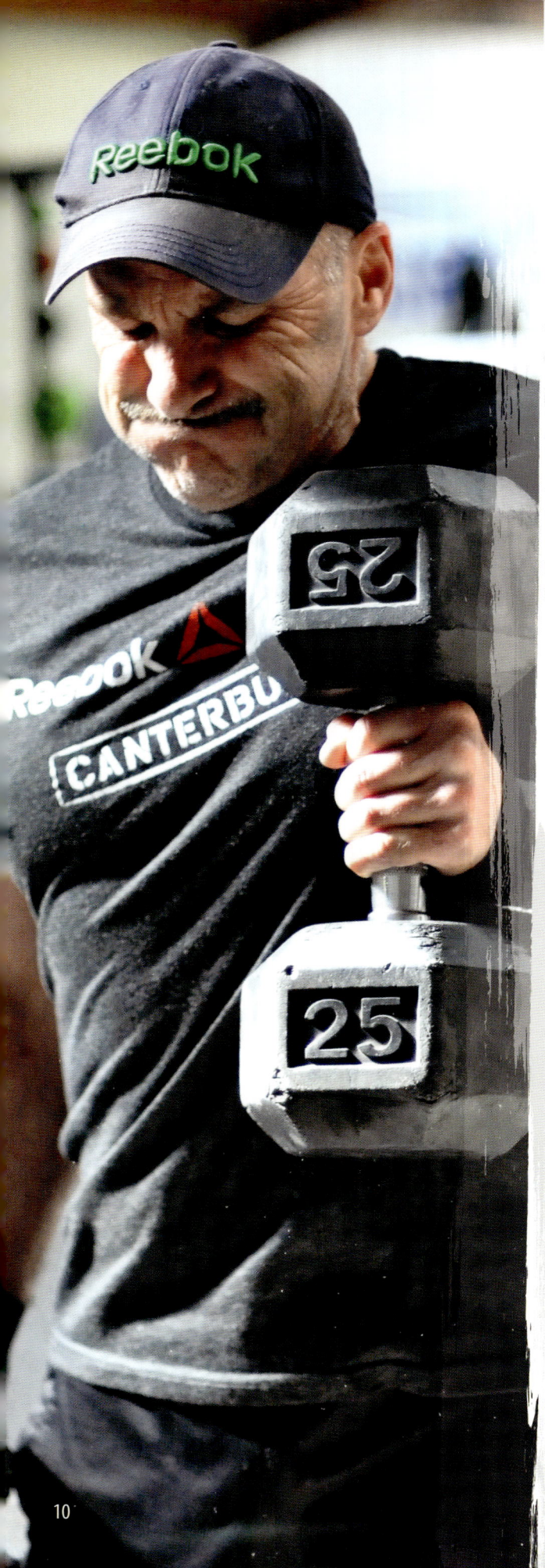

Even getting some of our guys doing half of what Ben and Owen do is a huge step forward.'

So how did two softly spoken, well-mannered young men who spent a lot of their early rugby days as the smallest guy in every front row they played in reach the pinnacle of All Black rugby, both members of the team that brought the World Cup home in 2011?

Sentimentalists will be pleased to know they do come from a rural, quintessentially Kiwi background.

Their father Ken, who has a major role to play in their success, was born in Motueka. His father was a fisherman, and Ken followed in his footsteps, taking up a fishing cadetship when he left school.

His work took him to Guam, working on an American boat, a super seiner, a giant vessel capable of carrying over 400 tonnes of tuna in a refrigerated hold. When he returned to Motueka he discovered his parents had moved to Australia.

He soon followed, and then joined the Australian Navy, at first in the Fleet Air Arm, and then as a submariner, working in electrical technical propulsion, based in Melbourne. Ken signed on for five years, and Ben was born in Melbourne in March 1984.

But Ken's career, and his life, almost ended off the coast of New South Wales.

'There was a big accident,' says Ken. 'When you come out of refit, and the submarine's been done up, you have to do a whole lot of tests, and the last test you do is a deep dive.

'We did that and got down to 800 feet, and a pipe burst. At that depth you've got a lot of water coming in and sea water in the batteries lets off a lot of gas. So we had breathing masks on.

Father Ken Franks going hard at the Reebok CrossFit Canterbury gym.

'When you do an emergency surface they pull back on the controls, and if you don't keep the sub dead square it starts to lean over. Then the pressure of the water can blow the sub over and over.

'The key figure is 90 degrees. If the sub gets over that water starts to flood in, the air rushes out, the tanks fill up, and you sink. We got to about 80 degrees and our engine fell off its mount, but we were able to get to the surface. At that point I was ready to leave.'

Ken heard that Talley's were building a big factory ship, so a return to Motueka was soon on the cards.

Owen was born in Motueka just before Christmas in 1987. A sister, Kate, would

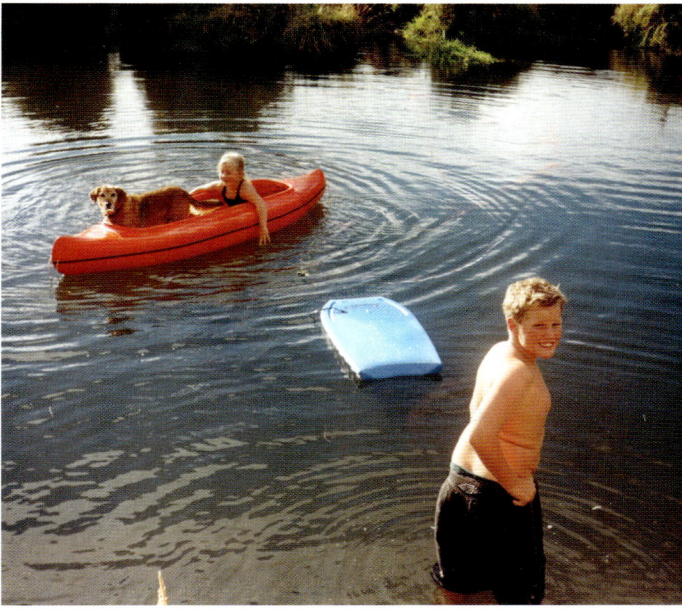

. . . . we were always playing rugby or cricket. Just typical small-town kids growing up.

complete the family four years after Owen was born.

For two boys who loved sport and the outdoors, life in Motueka was sweet.

'From what I hear about other brothers,' says Ben, 'some of them don't do anything together, whereas Owen and I have always got on pretty well from an early age.

'We spent most of our spare time outdoors. There were computer games and so on when we were growing up, but we didn't get into that too much. We had Nintendo at one stage, but that only lasted about two or three days – there was too much fighting.

'We lived in town, but Nana and Granddad had a pretty big property, and the family's always been into motorsport – Uncle Darren was NZ 250cc production road bike racing

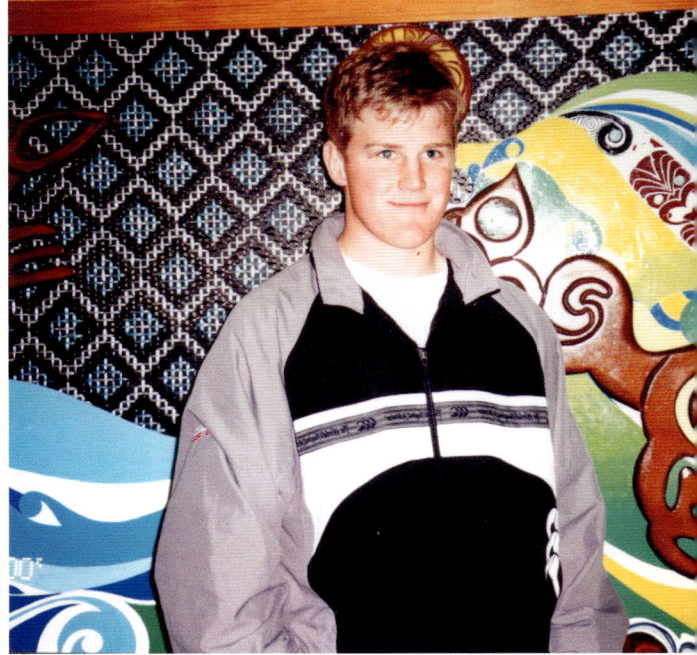

Top: Owen, aged 10, swimming with sister Kate.
Bottom: Ben in 2000.

11

champion. Granddad built us a go-kart one Christmas.

'As well as motorsport we were always playing rugby or cricket. Just typical small-town kids growing up. We loved fishing, and when Dad was working we'd be fishing off the Motueka wharf.'

At sport they were, Ken recalls, basically much like any other kid on the block. 'As a little boy Ben was a bit more coordinated than Owen. If you go back to midgets football Ben knew which way to run, but with Owen it was more a fifty-fifty call which direction he was going to go.'

Owen's earliest memories are playing for the Motueka Tigers league team when he was about five or six. His father was helping with the coaching. He endorses his father's memory of his early footy career. 'I remember tackling my own team-mates and people not being very happy with me. I forgot my boots once and Dad made me play in gumboots, which was quite embarrassing.'

At this stage, to be brutally honest, neither boy would have been a talent scout's first pick as a future All Black. Ben recalls himself as a 'chubby little kid' while Owen says he never considered himself much of a natural athlete.

But one thing they both enjoyed from the start was tackling. Ben started out in rugby as a six-year-old, but it was touch only and, 'I didn't like it too much because I couldn't get involved.'

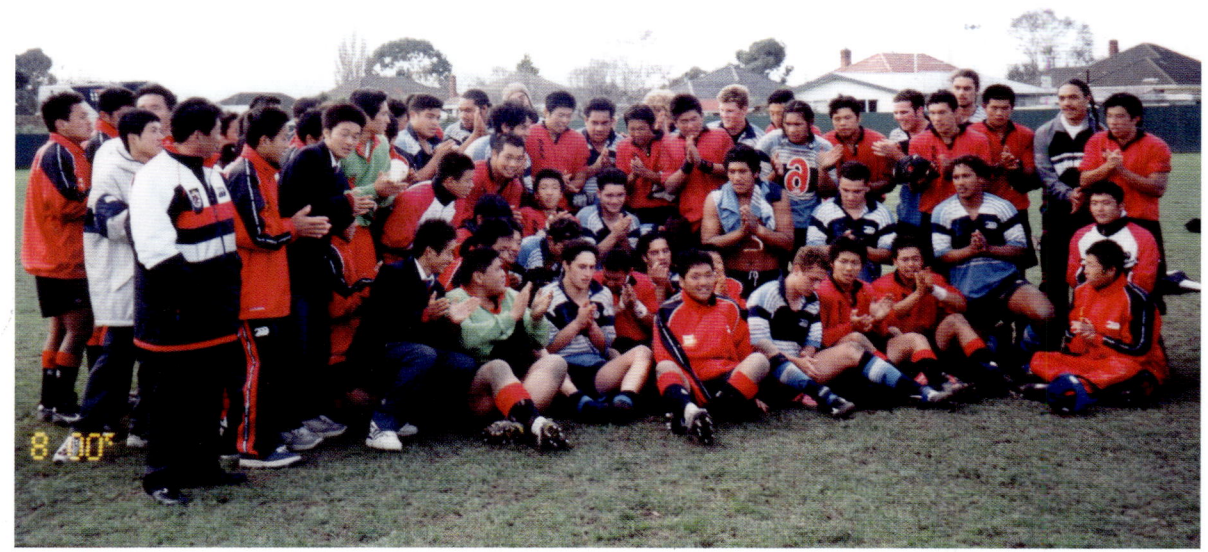

Above: Ben, featured back row middle, on tour in Japan with his high school First XV rugby team.
Right: Ben catching a 170 kg clean at Eastside Barbell, Christchurch, in 2011.

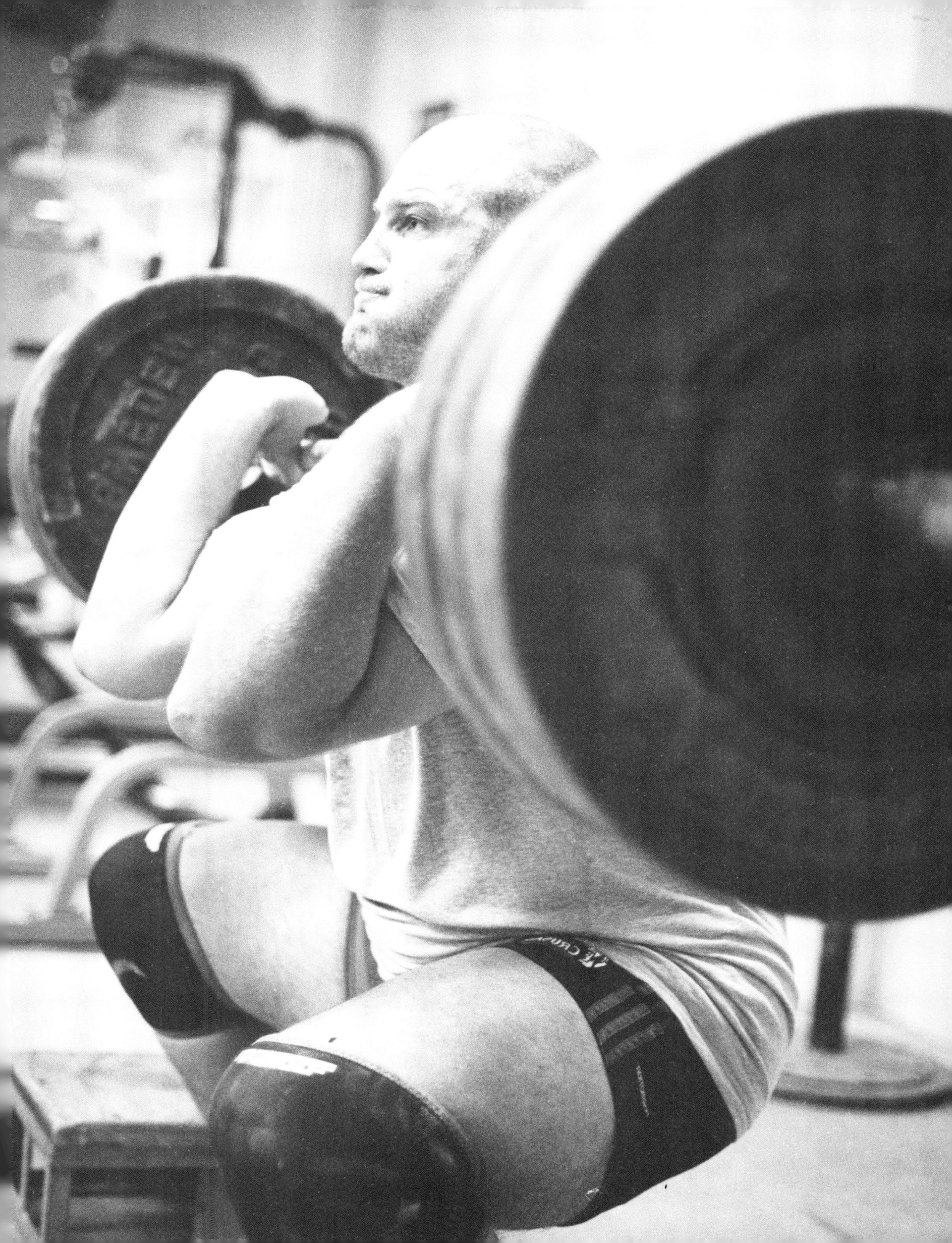

Owen says, 'I've always loved tackling as long as I can remember.' When the family moved to Christchurch 'I was playing for Lyttelton when I was 10 or 11, and it was always a competition to see who could do the biggest tackle, between me and my best friend in the team.

'Before a game Dad would look for the biggest player in the opposition team, who was usually an Island kid with a moustache. He'd say, "I want you to put a big tackle on him." Most times I would.'

The move to Christchurch, when Ben was starting his high school years, might have been a boost to Ben's budding rugby career. He'd made rep teams in Motueka. But in the big smoke those age-group achievements didn't seem to mean much.

'When we first came down from Mot,' says Ken, 'we knew that for rugby Boys' High was the school to be at in Christchurch, but they weren't interested. Hillmorton High School took us and Ben made the Canterbury under-14s from there. The next year he got into Boys' High.'

But although Ben's puppy fat had long since disappeared with weight training, after two years at Boys' High it was clear he wasn't likely to make the school's First XV.

A turning point came in the form of Aranui High School, which since 1997 had run a successful sports academy, and had rattled the cages of the traditional Christchurch rugby powerhouse schools by turning

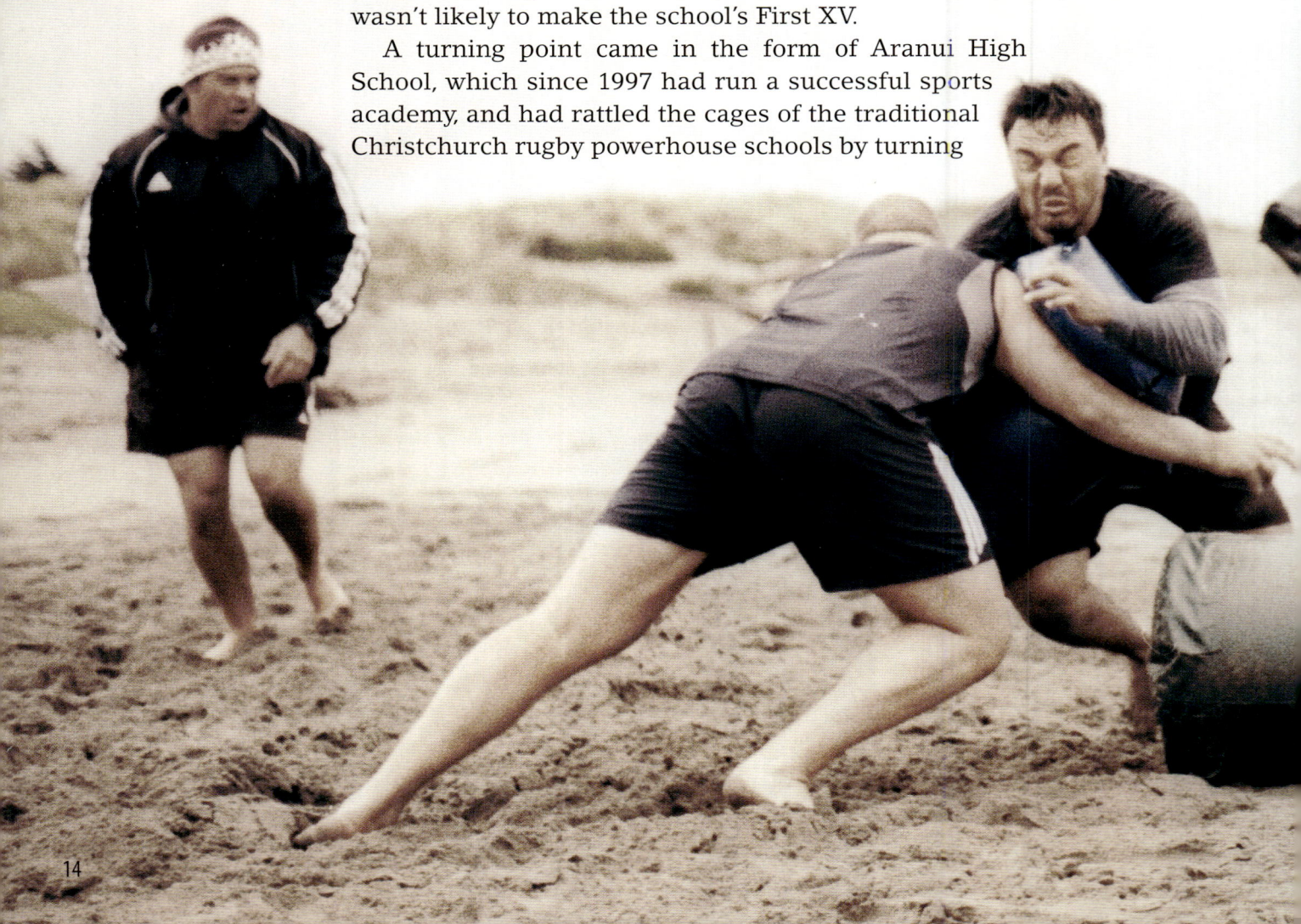

a lot of attention from the league the school had usually concentrated on to First XV rugby.

'Dad knew John Rangihuna who ran the Aranui Sports Academy,' says Ben. 'It sounded pretty good to me. You worked in the classroom for half the day and trained the rest. They were going on a tour to Japan too. I went over to Aranui, I loved it, and I made the Canterbury age-group teams.

'I wasn't very big. My first year at Aranui I was 85 kg and the other front-rowers were 130 kg and 140 kg. I wasn't that strong, although I was doing weights, so my technique had to be very good to survive.'

If he wasn't a giant by front-row standards, Ben didn't have small ambitions.

As a 13-year-old, he told his father, after they'd been to a Crusaders game, that he wanted to have a crack at being a professional player.

'We sat down,' says Ken, 'and I said, "Well, when everyone else is playing cricket in summer, you need to be in the gym or running."

'We figured that it was almost like an apprenticeship, from 13 to 18. By the time you get to 18 you're still immature from a rugby-playing perspective, but if you've been training for five years, you're not immature from the training perspective.

Owen hitting the tackle bags at Waimairi Beach during the 2011 rugby off season. People came from all over town to both hold and be the tackle bag while Ben and Owen used their holidays to hone their skills and conditioning.

'Ben bought into that and between the two of us we researched stuff, looking at things, and trying what looked like it'd work. I'm a big believer that you don't have to be the expert in everything, so we sought out who would show Ben the correct technique in lifting and so forth.'

Meanwhile kid brother Owen liked the look of what Ben was up to. 'I was probably annoying to Ben, because I wanted to hang out with him and his older friends, rather than my friends. That's been the case throughout our lives, with me always tagging along and doing what Ben was doing. As we got older that transferred in many ways into training and rugby.

'I was always a reasonable size when I was younger, but as I started getting into my teenage years, especially as a prop, I was smaller than a lot of the guys around me.

'Everything I have now all comes through the work I've done in the gym, and out on the training field. If I hadn't done that I think I'd just be a regular club player. I don't think I'd be that fast, or that strong, at all.

'The work had to happen. I realised, and Dad did too, when I first went to high school [Christchurch Boys' High School], that if we didn't really put the work in, we weren't going to get that far.

'That's why we trained so hard at such a young age, to try to get ahead of the rest of the group, because if we didn't do that training we would have just fallen behind.

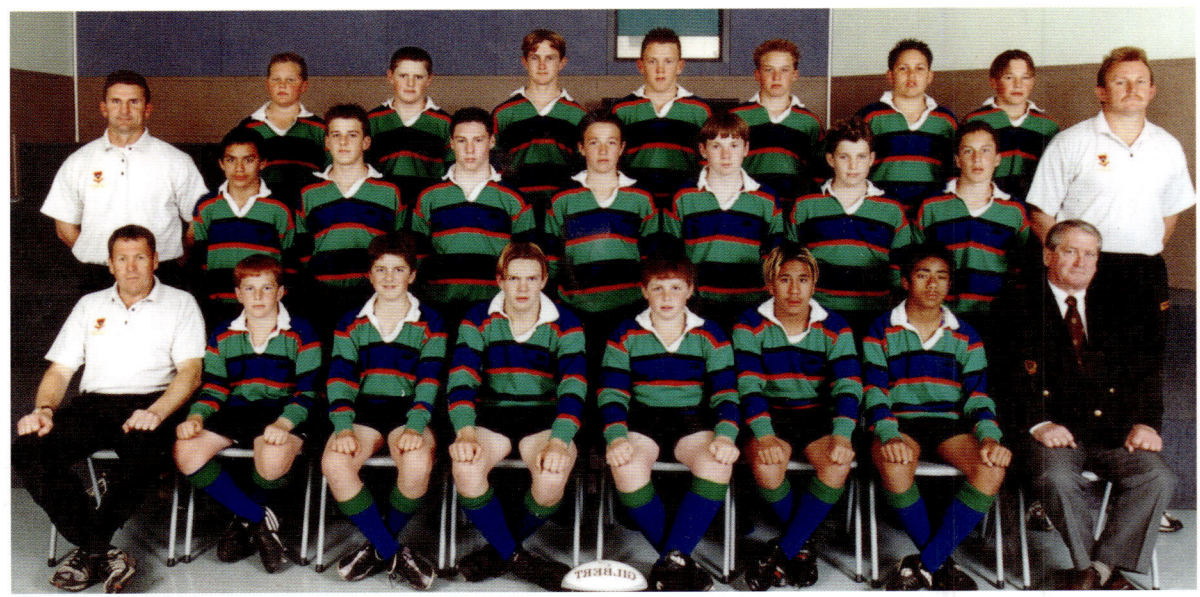

Young Owen Franks (back row far left) with his under 65 kg team.

'I've always thought it was pretty easy for me, because Ben was paving the way with Dad at training, and when he started getting the rewards by making rep teams, I was four years behind and I could see how his hard work was paying off.

'In my mind all I had to do was follow what he was doing, and look at the way he played, and pretty much do the same. So it was always a clear path for me.'

Weight training was always the ace up Ben and Owen's sleeves. They were coached in technique by experts. One was Warren Thin, a weightlifter and champion bodybuilder.

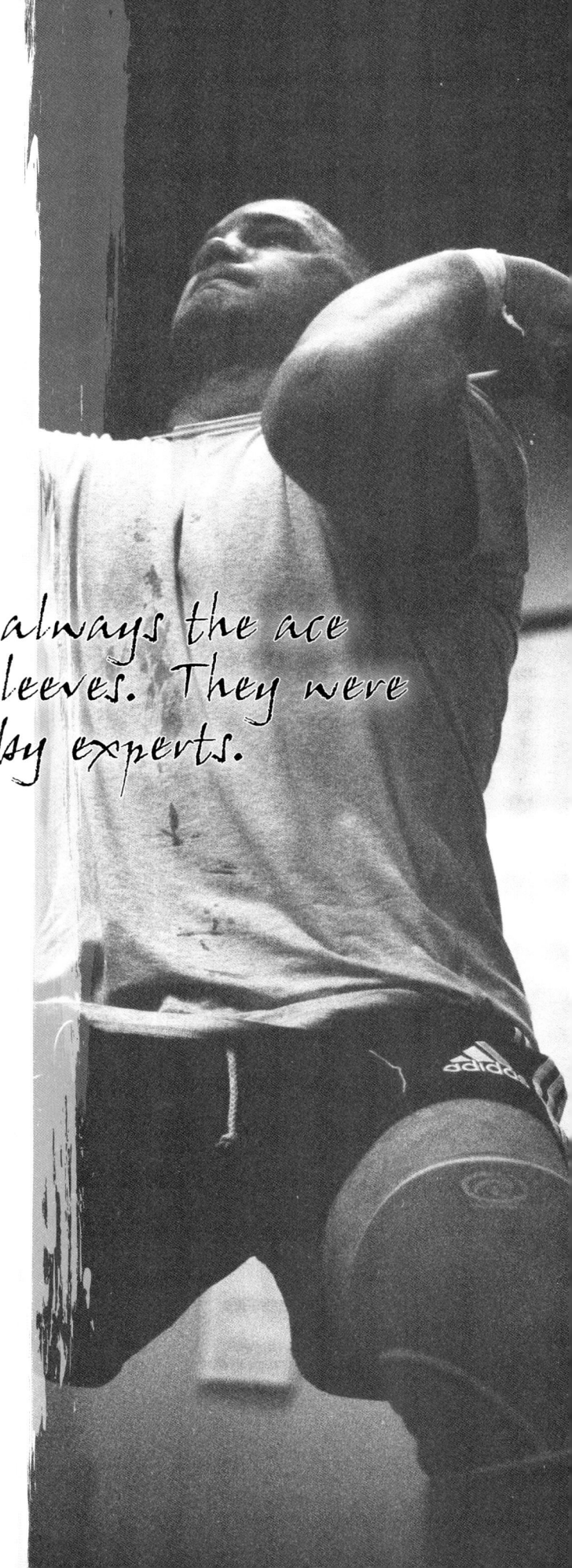

> *Weight training was always the ace up Ben and Owen's sleeves. They were coached in technique by experts.*

'Warren had been a professional at a higher level,' says Ben. 'So every time we did weight sessions it wasn't really just about weights. He'd be in my head about pushing myself, and with Dad he'd encourage me to think about what I was eating.

'It was a whole package of things – to be successful in any sport you have to tick all the same boxes.

'We knew that you have to start at a reasonable level and make the increases in weights gradual. It's a process and you have to be patient.

'I still work with Warren now. We discuss what I think I need to be better at for my game, and he suggests what the exercises should be, and how to go about it.

'I say what the results I'd like to see on the field are, and we work from there. There's a lot of trust between us.

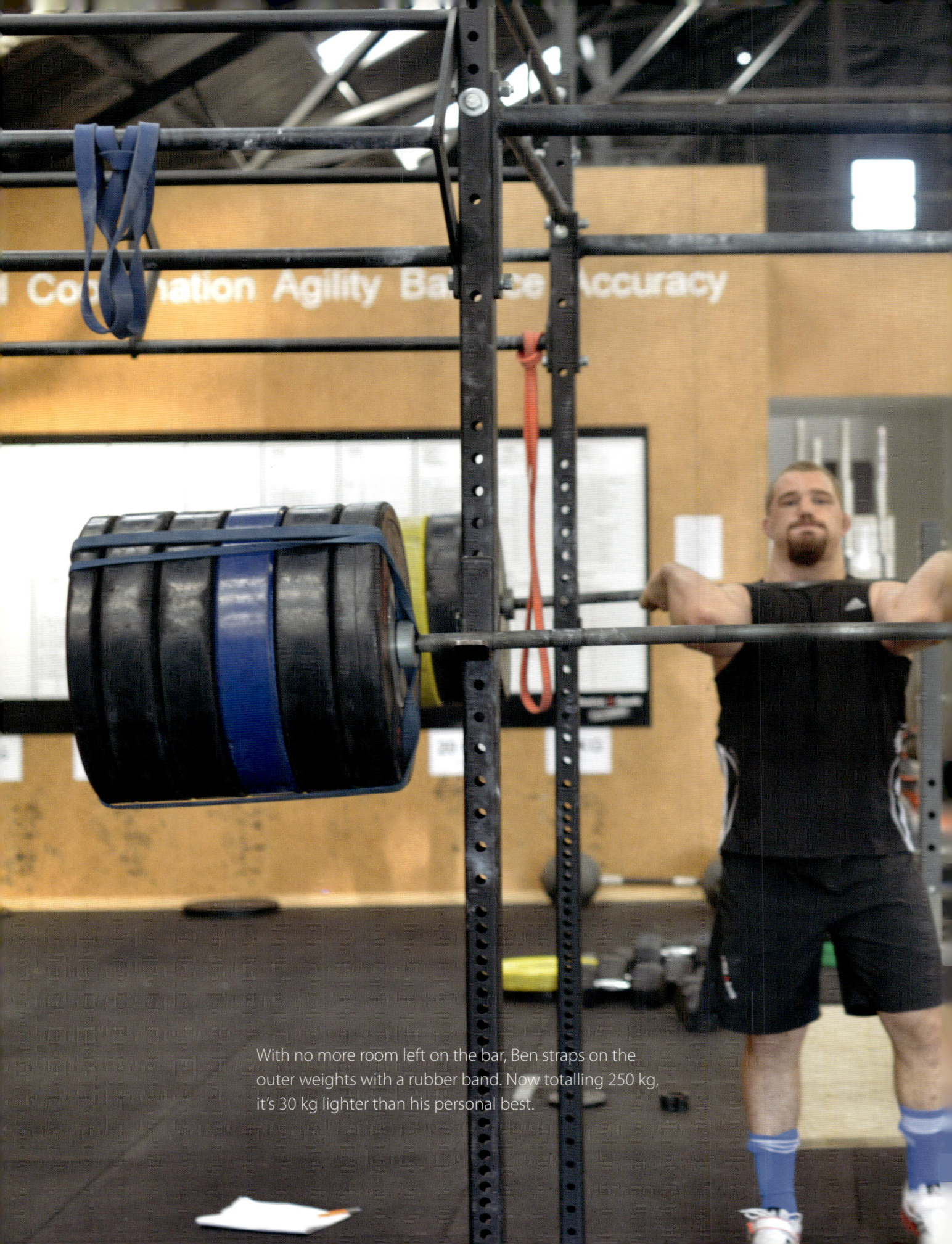

With no more room left on the bar, Ben straps on the outer weights with a rubber band. Now totalling 250 kg, it's 30 kg lighter than his personal best.

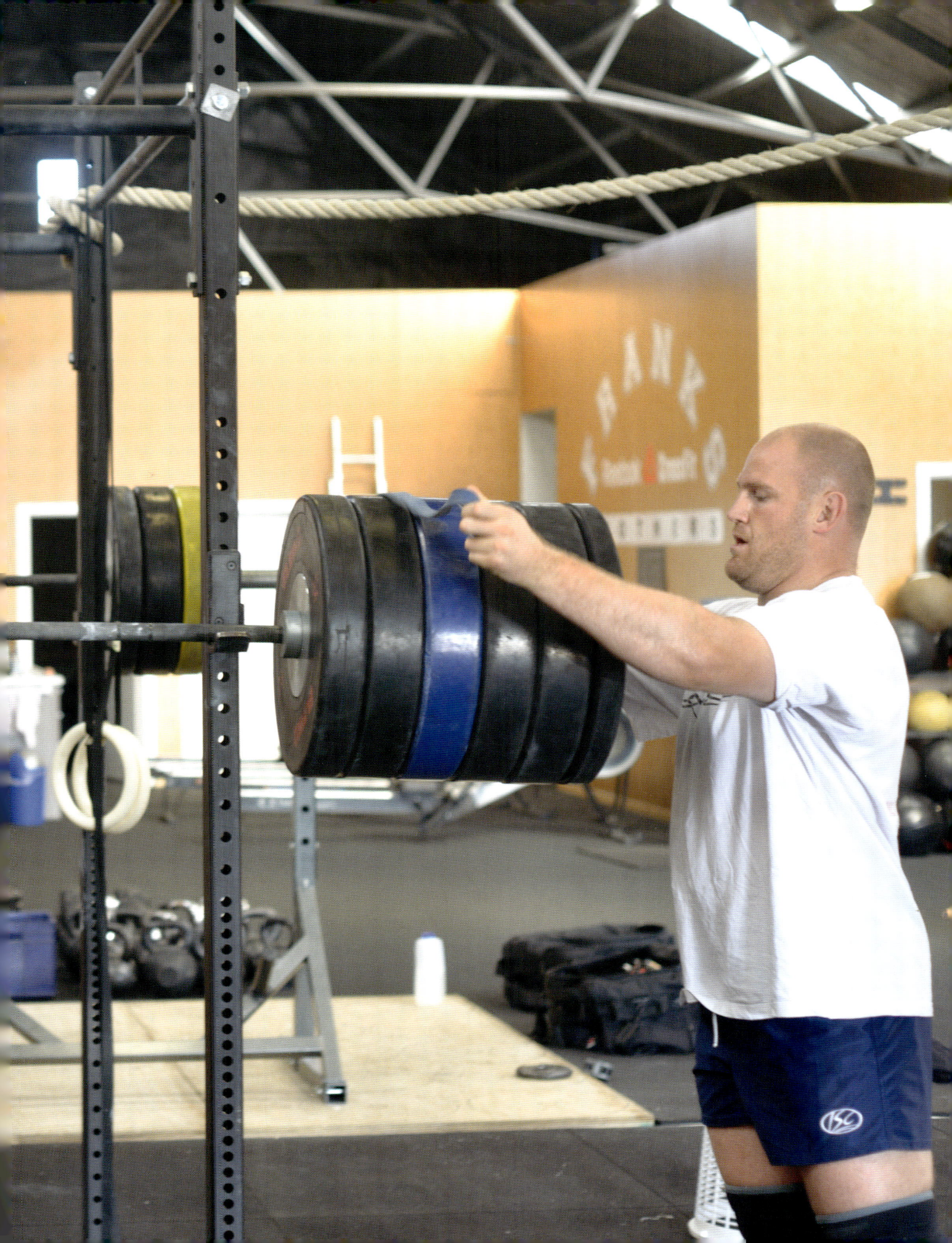

'People see the weights Owen and I lift now, but they don't see the five, six, seven years we spent working up to that, in small steps.' The Franks, says Ken, have a philosophy of technique before weight. 'The weight will come.'

Ken says he's 'a big fan for not reinventing the wheel, but I am keen to find out what's being done in your field now.

'So we'd look on the internet and we identified that the NFL had big guys who were so fast over 40 yards. So then we started to find out why they were able to do that, and started to introduce the way they trained into what we were doing.

'We were looking for the things that worked for us. Sometimes they were rubbish, but other times there were methods that did work for the boys.'

Nutrition was one area where the Franks gained a reputation for being massively disciplined. Colin Meads jokes that 'if only people like myself, Bunny Tremain and Waka Nathan had known we shouldn't eat bacon and eggs on game day, think how good we might have been.'

There are so many different diets and theories on what you should eat; I just try to keep it as simple as I can.

Pinetree might be pleased to hear that the diets Ben and Owen stick to are not as New Age as is sometimes reported.

Owen laughs at suggestions they live on spirulina shakes and silverbeet sandwiches. 'There are so many different diets and theories on what you should eat; I just try to keep it as simple as I can. Oats for breakfast, eggs, meat, fish, chicken, wraps for lunch, a lot of fruit.

'We try to keep it straightforward. It's pretty simple. Some people get caught up, but I think the more you keep it basic the better off you'll be.

'When I'm training a lot, working really hard pre-season, I'm just eating as much as I can. I have a pretty fast metabolism, so I lose weight very quickly, and can put it on very quickly.

'I know my body pretty well, and off season I know how much training I'm doing, and what I need to eat. But I'm not fanatical about food 24/7. I just try to keep it clean, and avoid processed foods.'

Attention to detail and hard training started to pay off when Ben was still a teenager. Selection in Canterbury under-16, and then

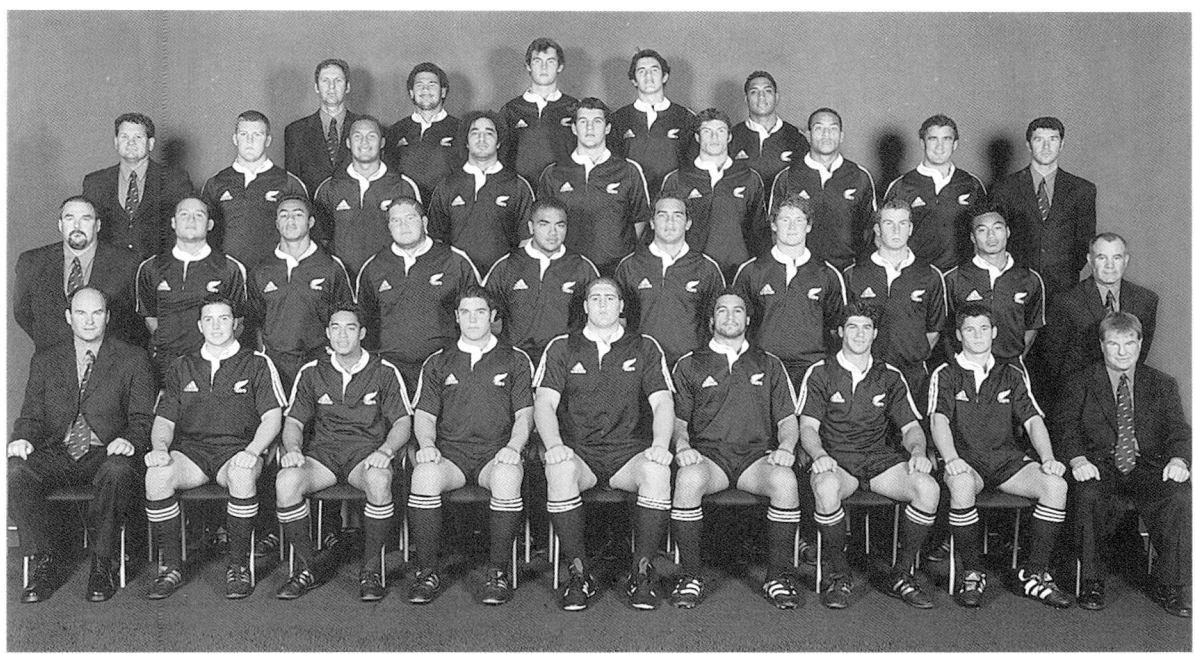

The 2003 NZ Under-19 side. Ben is in the third row, second from the left.

Canterbury under-19, sides led to him making the New Zealand under-19 team in 2003, travelling to France for the world junior championship. New Zealand made the final, but lost to South Africa.

'Even though I'd make the teams,' says Ben, 'I was usually the guy who wasn't expected to make it. I was the guy at the trials who wasn't the automatic choice, so I always tried to work harder. It's always been second nature to try to do extra stuff.

'Out of school I went to the Canterbury [Rugby] Academy for a couple of years before I was professional. I did some labouring jobs, and I went up and did a scallop season with some family friends. I basically did stuff that worked out well with my training.'

There were differences in the way the Franks family approached things even then. Ken says, 'I remember they used to have three big anchor chain links at Rugby Park. You were supposed to grab hold of them and drag them.

'Ben was at the academy and we came down and got a sprint harness, and tied a rope from the back of the harness to the chain, got down in a propping position and dragged it that way. They'd be wondering what the hell we were doing.

'We've had a few battles with the rugby union, saying to them don't just judge the boys on their age. Judge them on their playing ability, or their training ability.

'Don't tell them they can't do this because they're 18, when they may have been training to get to that level for four or five years.'

Ben recalls that 'at the start there were times when it was extremely difficult. I'd been doing weights and running hills and heaps of different stuff, but when I turned up when I was 18 you have different people wanting you to do stuff. They all have a different opinion. I just knew what worked for me, and I butted heads with quite a few people. But I stuck at it, and it got me to where I am now.

'In a rugby squad you've got about 30 guys. For me, I'm trying to get myself to the next level, so I can perform for the team. When you've got a trainer looking after 30 guys, he's looking at a more general goal.

'Weights for me has never been about getting strong, it's about how it'll affect my technique for rugby, so I've always wanted to know, "Why am I doing this exercise? What am I doing this for?"

'I can understand how that could be annoying, but I just wanted to know the reason for everything. If they gave me a reason and I understood it, then I'd buy into it fully. Everything had to have a reason, or otherwise I'd do something else.

Steam rises off John Afoa, Ben and Jerome Kaino during an All Black training session in Edinburgh, 2008. This was Ben's first All Black tour.

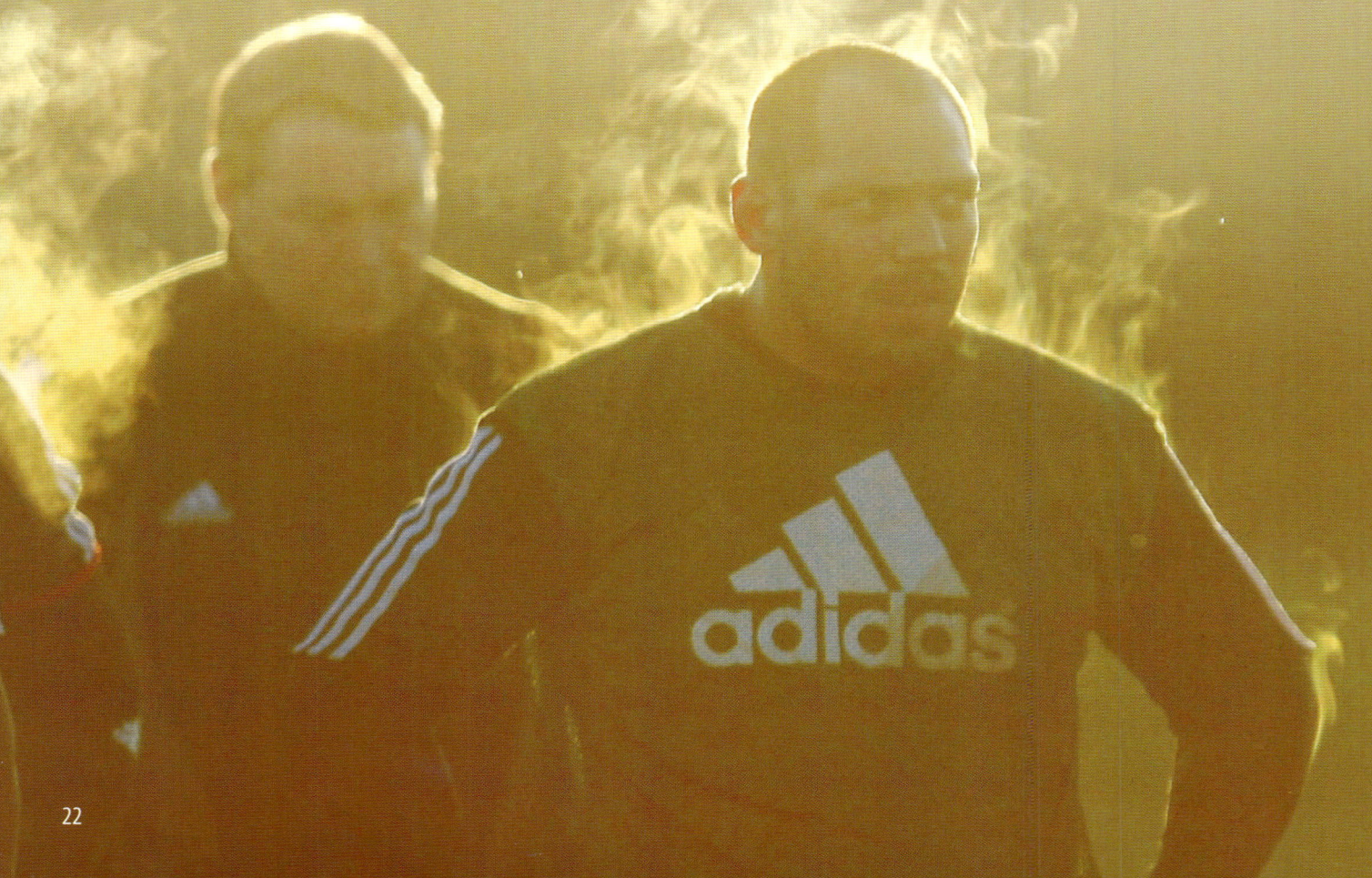

'Rugby's not a generic sport, so weight training can't be the same for everyone. What I do is a lot different to what a lock does. I may do things a lot differently to what another prop might do. My needs could be the total opposite to those of another prop.

'Rugby now is a cut-throat sport, especially at the academy stage, where you're with a big bunch of guys and you're trying to pop your head up above the rest.

'If you really want it you have to find a way to put yourself ahead of the pack. It's not about being selfish – it's about trying to make it.

'Some players don't realise that until it's too late, and they find they're not there.

'I found that in the New Zealand under-19 team. I look at the photo from that team from 2003, and only three out of 26 are still playing for the All Blacks – myself, Liam Messam and Hosea Gear. Only six out of 26 played for the All Blacks at all. And that's from a group who were considered some of the best young players in the country at the time.

'I had a dream that I might be an All Black when I was a little kid, like every kid in a backyard playing made-up games.

'When I started to get serious the path was a series of steps. I made a Canterbury under-16 team; then it was making New Zealand under-19. When I made the Crusaders, in 2006, in the first year I didn't get many starts. The next season I started all the time, and then the season after that I thought, "I think I can be an All Black."

'In 2008 after Super Rugby I didn't get picked for the Tri Nations, but during the NPC I went up to the All Black camps three or four times, so I knew that I had a bit of a shot. I was named for the end-of-year northern tour. I didn't get a test on that tour, but I played in the midweek Munster game, which I loved.'

While brother Ben was working his way towards the Crusaders, Owen was basically following in his bootsteps. Like Ben, he arrived with a real training ethic.

'We'd always done a lot of sit-ups and press-ups, and I think I was 14 when Dad bought me my first gym membership to QEII, and I started weight training. Dad never pushed us to lift heavy weights when we started; it was all about technique.

'We were lucky enough to meet a guy called Lee Attrill, who is a former Olympic weightlifter, and he's always been huge on technique before weight and making sure the body's moving how it should be.

'He put me and Ben in good stead, learning how to squat properly, and doing all the main exercises correctly.'

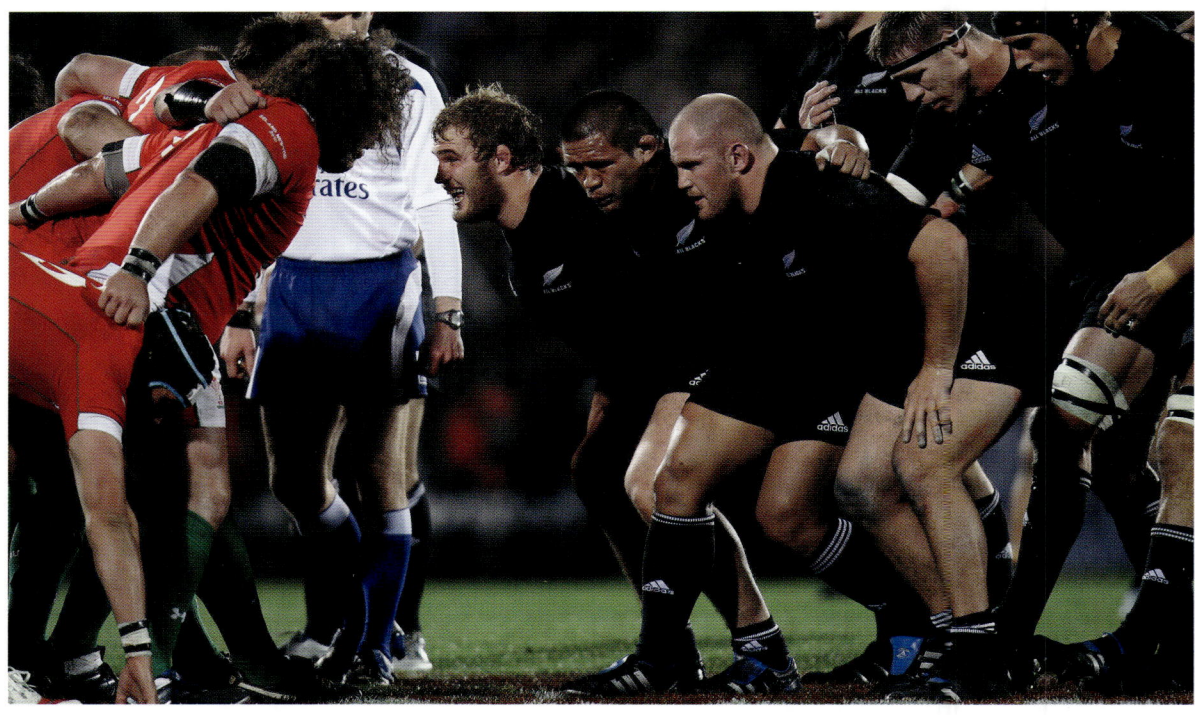

Owen and Ben were the All Blacks' starting props for the first test between New Zealand and Wales at Dunedin in 2010. Keven Mealamu is the hooker.

Owen went to Christchurch Boys' High, where he played hooker before switching to prop fulltime.

'When I settled into prop I played both sides of the front row almost all the way through. My first year in the First XV I played both sides, but then in my last year at high school I played tighthead all year.'

His obvious talent took him into the New Zealand secondary schools team of 2005 that toured Australia, and in his first year out of school he was playing senior rugby for Linwood, as a loosehead prop. The next year he decided it was time to concentrate on being a tighthead.

For both Ben and Owen, technique in the scrum has been crucial. As strong as they are now they say there were many years when they couldn't rely on size or brute strength to get them through.

Living in Canterbury they had the man they call 'the scrum doctor', Mike Cron, to learn from. Cron, a former prop himself, has been with the All Blacks coaching staff since 2004, but he also runs numerous coaching clinics for young props.

'Mike Cron's scrum sessions started when I was only 16 or 17,' says Ben, 'although not on a regular basis. Mike showed me what

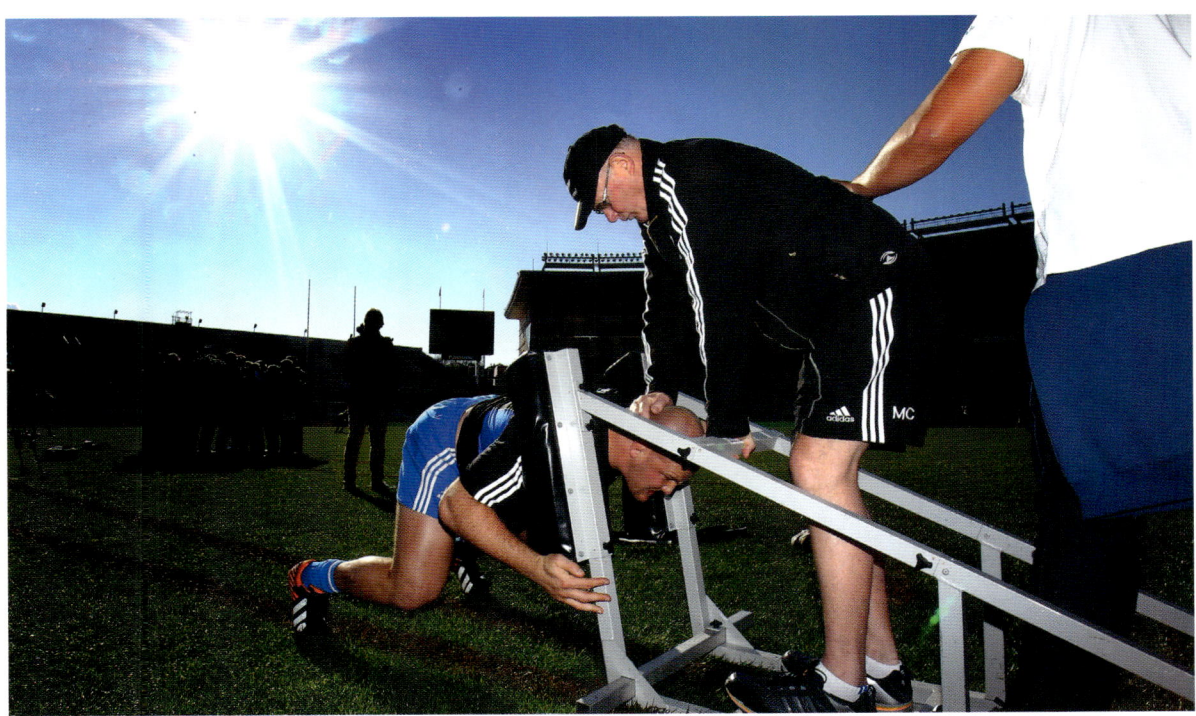

Ben training with scrum guru Mike Cron during the captain's run prior to the All Blacks' match against Australia at Eden Park in 2012.

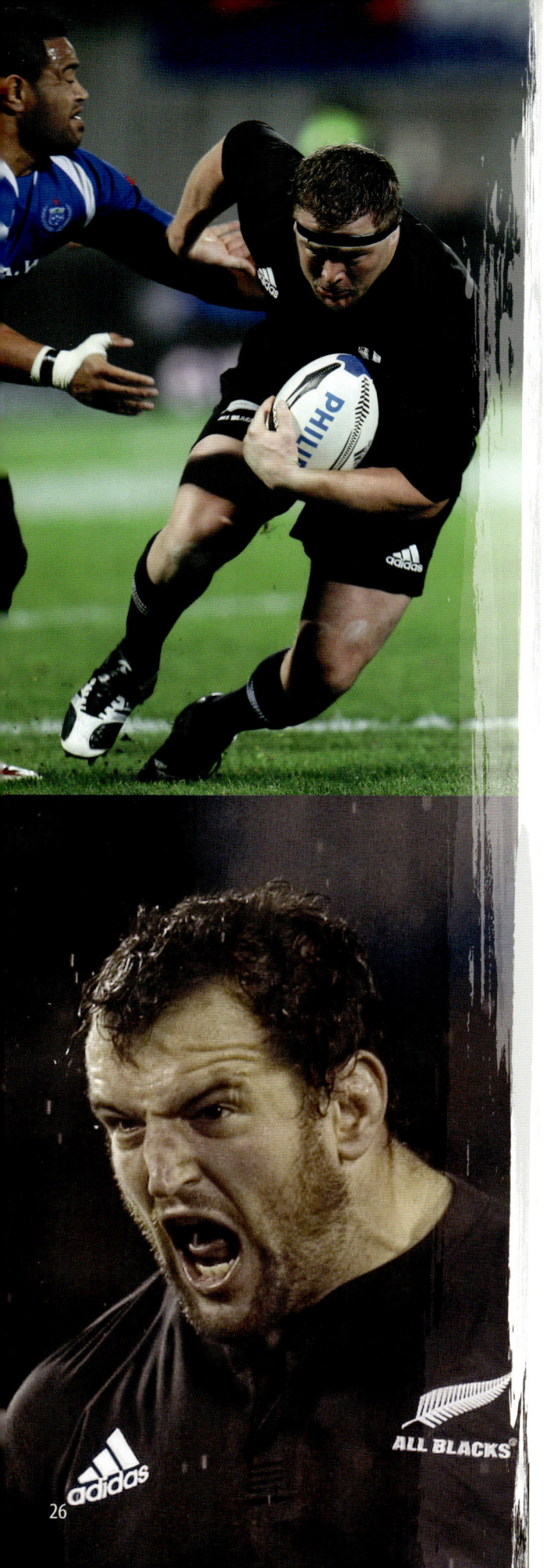

I should do, and I did a lot of repetitions at home, some of them in front of a mirror.

'As the years have gone on my technique has been an evolving thing, working to keep improving.'

For Owen, learning scrum skills started with his father. 'When they first started doing live scrums in the rugby I was playing, I guess I was about 10 or 11, Dad took me down to the garage, and basically taught me how to have a flat back, made me do a set-up in front of him, and told me when my back was flat and when it wasn't.

'Watching Ben was important too. Seeing guys like Greg Somerville was an influence, and then when Carl Hayman came onto the scene he was definitely someone I tried to model my technique on.

'I first met Mike Cron when I was about 16, and I've seen him at least once or twice every year at clinics and so on. He's not only been a prop himself, but he has the biomechanical knowledge behind everything he teaches. It's all proven stuff. So his influence has been big.'

Ben has propped for the All Blacks on both sides of the scrum – a remarkable feat when you consider how different the demands of the positions are.

'Shag [Steve Hansen] said to me in 2009 that if I wanted to be a permanent part of the All Blacks I was going to have to be the guy who could play both sides of the scrum. It wasn't an official sit-down, more a tap on the shoulder sort of thing.

'That really altered my mindset and the way I went about things, with the Crusaders too.

'I had to take three years to make sure I could play both sides to make the World Cup,

Ben and Owen were both influenced by top All Black props Greg Somerville (top) and Carl Hayman (left).

so I could be comfortable on either side. In the Crusaders in 2011 it got to a point with rotation in the front row that I was playing a different position each week, back and forth.

'I was in a competition with John Afoa and Neemia Tialata, and that definitely helped me get an edge.'

Owen, who has nailed down the tighthead jersey in the All Blacks, says, 'At loosehead you're being hit down on. The tighthead is almost hitting down on you, so you have to be really strong at taking the hit. You need a really strong neck and back.

'It's more of an attacking position. On your ball you have to get a good hit, but on the opposition ball it's really the loosehead's time to shine where he can disrupt, and make a menace of himself.

'As a tighthead, on your own ball you've got a lot of the responsibilities, because if you don't do your job the whole scrum can disintegrate, and you can be made to look pretty stupid.

'So it's more about technique, being sound, and being able to use your body well. Just being rock solid I guess.

'One of the keys at tighthead is to be able, if the scrum doesn't go well, to stick to your guns and keep doing what you know is going to work.

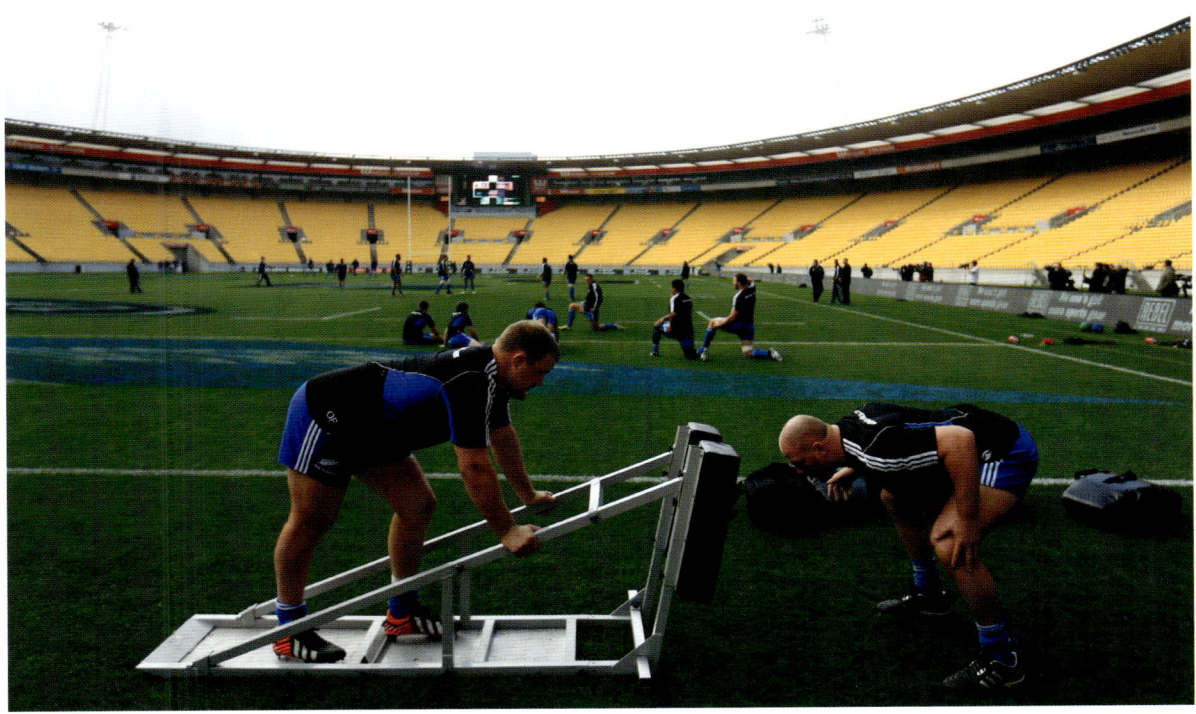

Owen (left) and Ben scrum training in Wellington, 2012.

'Sometimes you'll see a tighthead who has a bad scrum, and then he lacks a bit of confidence, and then he does something to compensate, and it just snowballs from there.

'It's about keeping calm and just being technically really good. On the opposition ball you're also trying to attack and help the loosehead disrupt.

'You do notice it when you've got a good tighthead lock behind you, because you have the power to explode through on the hit. You may get caught short with your legs underneath you on the hit, but you can still power out. But if you don't have a technically good lock behind you it makes it tough.'

Ben was the first to make the Crusaders, and when he was initially selected, in 2006, Robbie Deans was still coaching the team.

The Crusaders are famous for extensive work in the summer to form team unity, although Ben isn't certain that team bonding exercises is the main reason for the team's successes.

'It was my first experience [in 2006] at that level, so to me it was

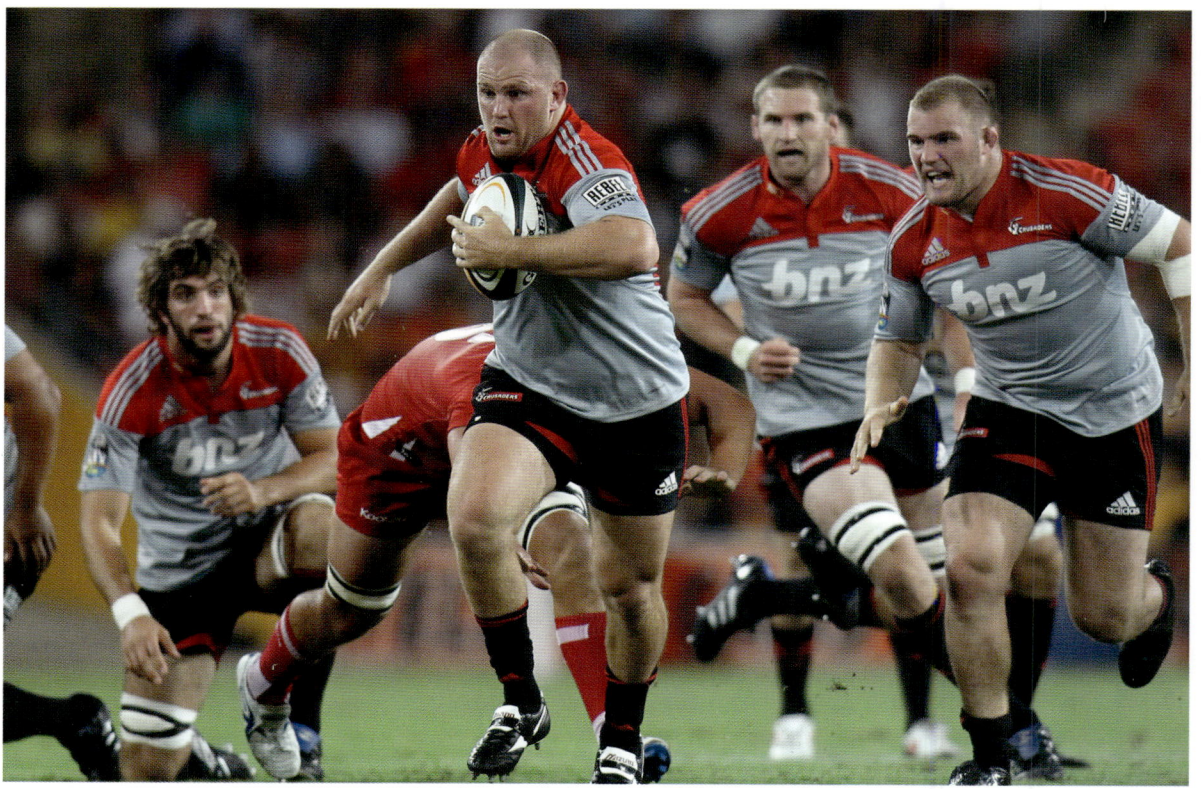

Ben leads a Crusaders raid with Kieran Read (middle) and Owen in close support during this Super match against the Reds at Brisbane, 2010.

just how it was done. We'd go away for three or four days locally, or go to Australia, and have meetings about the team culture. We'd have a theme for the year. I wouldn't say I really enjoyed it; I've always been a bit more of a doer than just talking about things.

'I always felt the success of the Crusaders was that there were 25 guys who truly wanted to win the competition. The Crusaders seem to attract those sorts of players. In a sport like rugby the team is obviously very important, because if you want to achieve your goals it won't matter how motivated you are as an individual, you won't get anywhere unless the team is firing as well.

'There is a difference between people just being there, and people who truly want to win, and that's when the Crusaders have been most successful, when there have been players with that attitude.

'I always remember John Rangihuna telling us at the [Aranui]

The All Blacks is an environment where you know there's rarely a second, much less a third, chance.

academy that attitude is everything, which comes from [league coach] Wayne Bennett.

'Dad used to say, "You never know who's watching", and that's even more true today. You look at some of the Super 15 squads, and there are guys who have been cut who never even got onto the field.

'Why have they been cut? They were judged at what they did at training, and what attitude they brought to it.'

If the competition is intense in Super Rugby, it goes up several notches in the All Blacks, says Ben.

'The All Blacks is an environment where you know there's rarely a second, much less a third, chance. You want to get it right straight away. You have the weight of the country's expectations on you as well.

'The people you're with are hugely motivated and you have experts there in every field working with you.

'It's hard to compare the All Black environment with the Crusaders or Canterbury because with the All Blacks the time you have before you play is so much shorter.

'In a way the All Blacks need to make things as streamlined as possible in the time they have, so as a player you're able to pick it up,

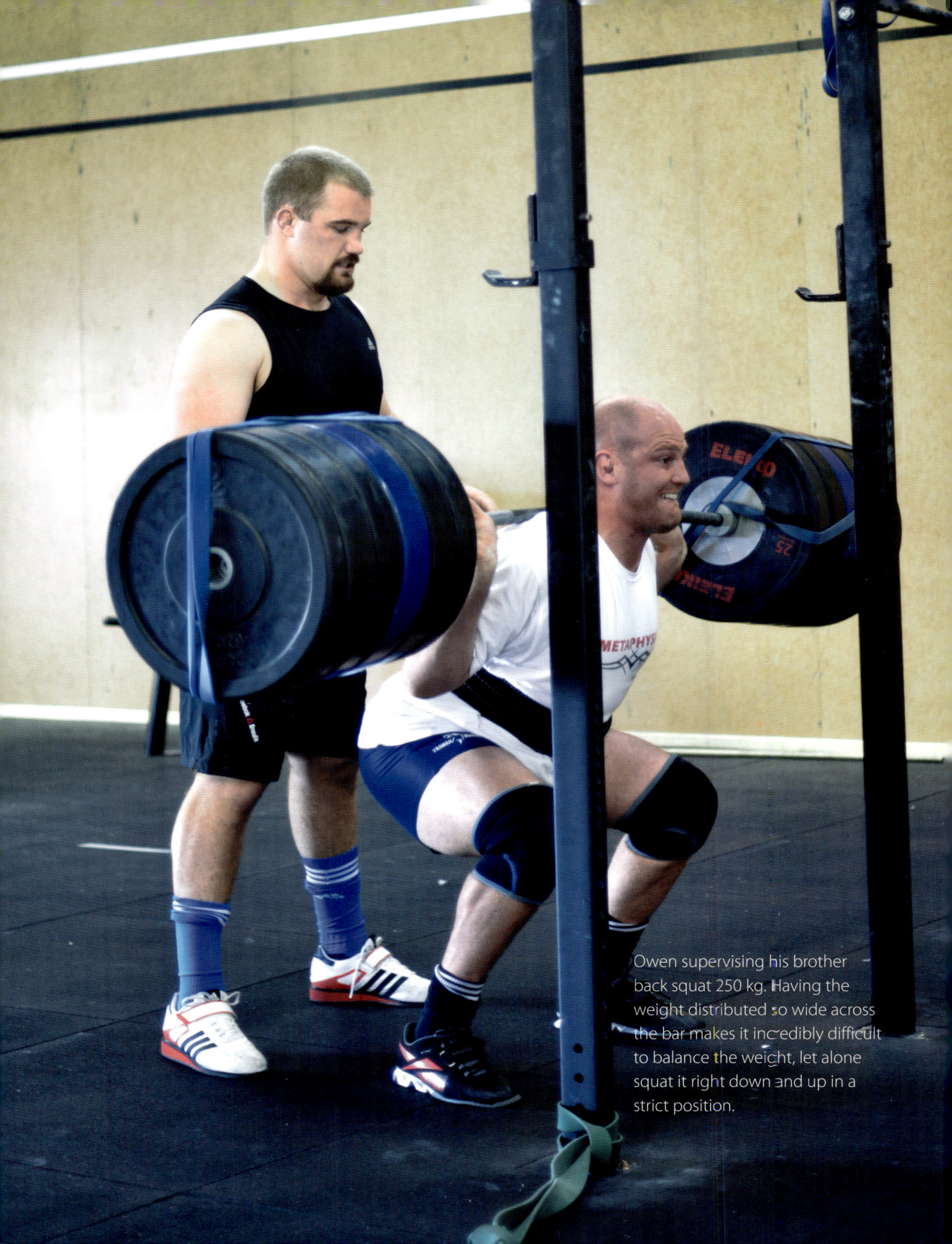

Owen supervising his brother back squat 250 kg. Having the weight distributed so wide across the bar makes it incredibly difficult to balance the weight, let alone squat it right down and up in a strict position.

and get comfortable with what's wanted straight away.

'With Super Rugby it's a big challenge to keep form for 18 weeks or more. The squads are bigger, there are injuries over that time, so you're in a very different position to the All Blacks.'

The front row, at any level, is a dark, scary mystery to anyone who has never played there, and the brothers say at international level, especially, there's no such thing as an easy day at the office.

'The good props come at you every scrum,' says Ben. 'The difference between a good day and a bad day in scrummaging is so small that I've never had a day where I've thought afterwards, "Gee, the scrums were easy today".'

Owen swears that 'as far as international props go, I can honestly say there's not one who is easier than the other.

'Every prop is different, every loosehead I've come up against has different strengths and weaknesses. The guys I play the most, like Benn Robinson from Australia, you develop quite a good battle with. Every time you play you want to outdo each other. I guess they're

Every prop is different, every loosehead I've come up against has different strengths and weaknesses.

going to be the toughest, because you know them so well, and have scrummed against them so much. Everyone is professional now, and no one wants to give an inch.

'At lower levels you may get the odd guy who's a bit easier, but once it comes to internationals there's not a lot of difference between most scrums.'

The height of their careers came in 2011 when they were both in the All Black squad that won the World Cup.

Ben says, not having been in the 2007 team eliminated in the infamous quarter-final in Cardiff, he was 'pretty much like every other New Zealander, I just wanted us to win it'.

The nation's expectations didn't weigh him down. 'I really enjoyed the whole experience. Usually it's not until we go overseas, to South Africa or France, that we strike crowds that are really noisy and get into the game. In New Zealand we're a lot quieter. You tend not to hear from the crowd until you do something bad.

'In the World Cup the flags were out, the crowds were excited, everyone was coming up and wishing you well. We all loved it.'

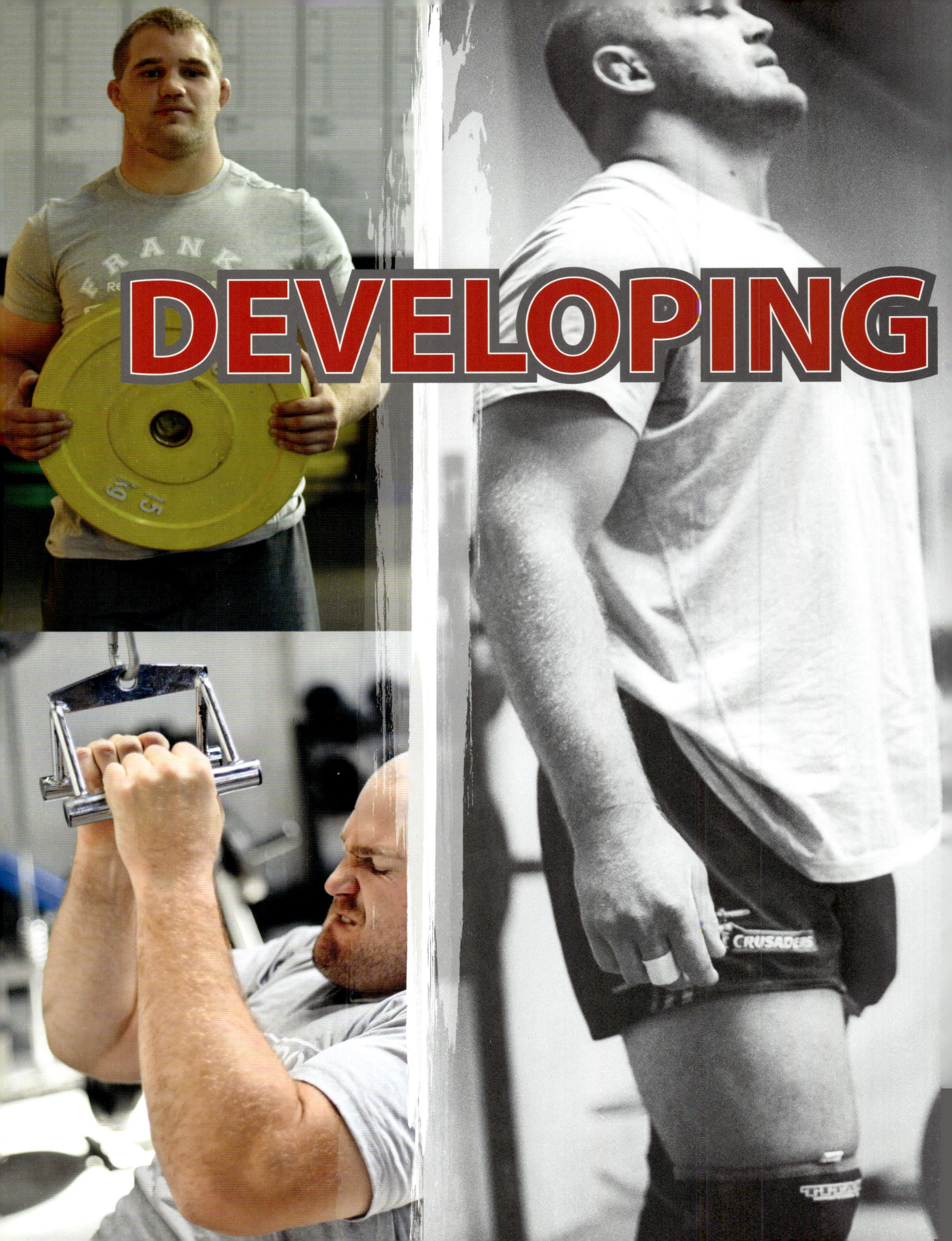

DEVELOPING

AN ATHLETE

The human body, like most living things, responds and adapts to its surrounding environment, rapidly evolving to whatever adversity it is exposed to. What goes into the body has a direct effect on its growth and output.

Much like a plant, if the body gets good nutrients, sunlight and is regularly watered it will grow well. If exposed to resistance, such as heavy winds, a plant will grow naturally stronger. The human body is not much different. However, unlike a tree or plant, the human body has many moving parts. Each part has a range of motion and measurable strength and endurance. At the core the body has 356 bones all connected together by ligaments. Tendons connect muscle groups to bones that combine to control the body's movements. Details get more complex as the heart muscle pumps blood around the body carrying oxygen and other necessities from the lungs and other origins.

When any of the body's functions are challenged they will grow stronger: mentally and physically. The secret, however, lies in regular practice developed by a determined routine. But contrary to the saying 'practice makes perfect', it is important to learn the correct methods. Perfect practice makes perfect. For example, learning the alphabet is advised before learning to read. Learning the correct movements is just as critical when learning to exercise, not to mention recovery and nutrition contributing more than half of the physical development over exercise itself.

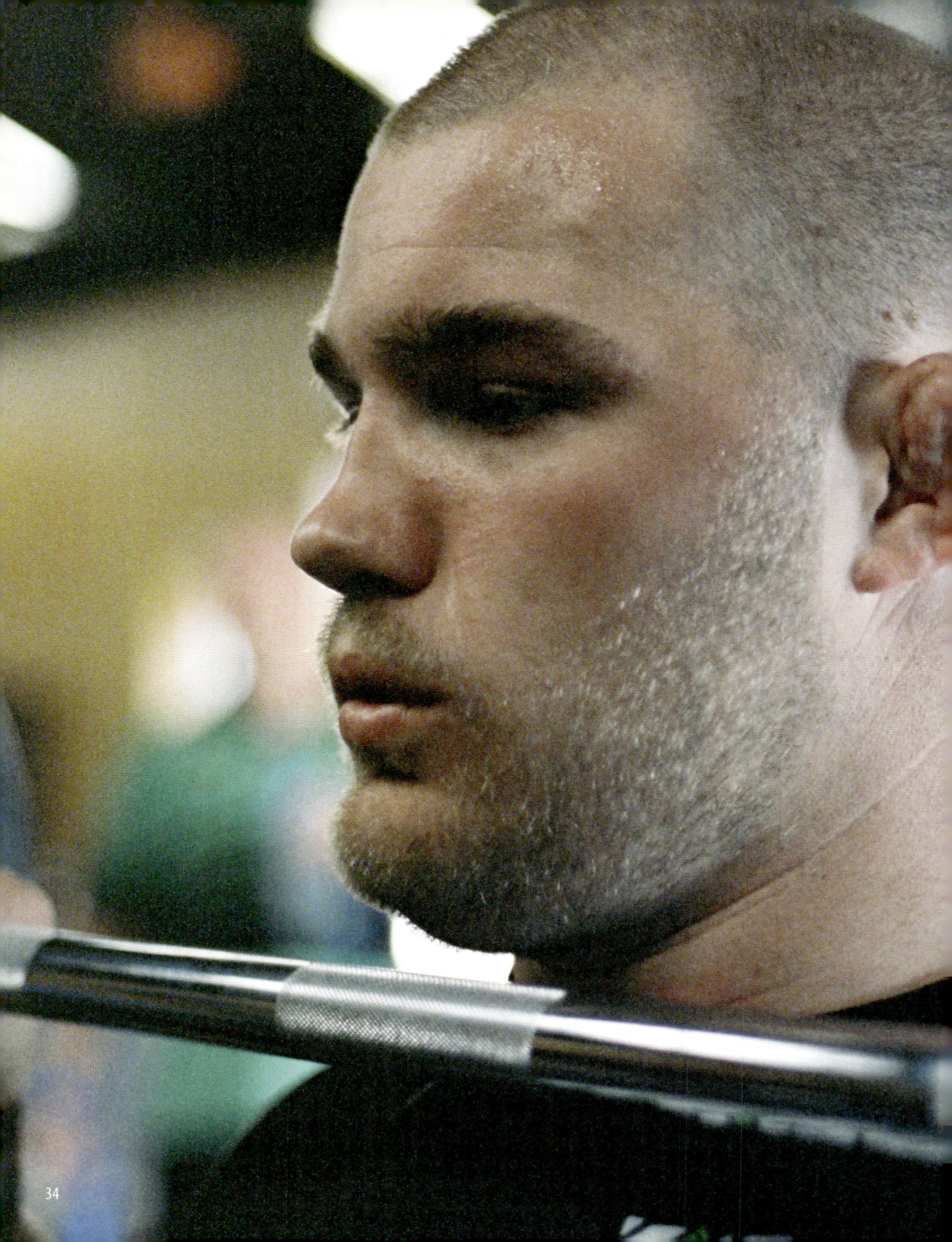

What ultimately separates a professional athlete from others is mental toughness. You can have all the speed, power and strength in the world, but that is useless if you can't bring it all together when it's required. This introduction to training has been developed not only by Ben and Owen Franks, but a collection of their favourite and most effective trainers and coaches. It will help young aspiring athletes set off in the right direction and develop the training habits required to grow into top-class competitors.

If you are already playing a club sport like rugby, soccer, basketball, etc, you may know that it is difficult to commit to a personal training schedule outside of your club commitments. Therefore the best opportunity to physically improve yourself is outside the regular season, known as the 'post-' and 'pre-' season.

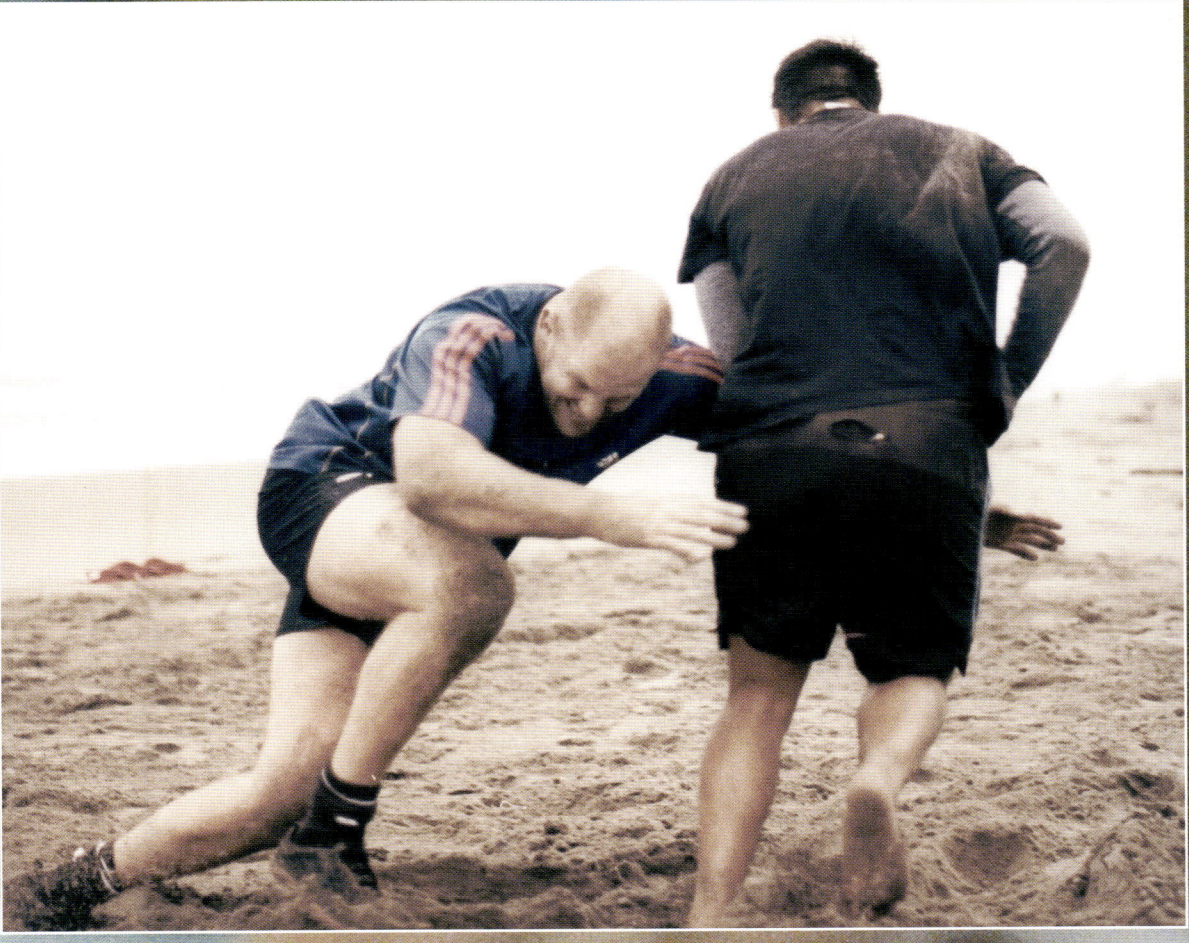

Above: Ben toughing it out on the beach with trainer Scott Hanson.
Left: Owen is all concentration.

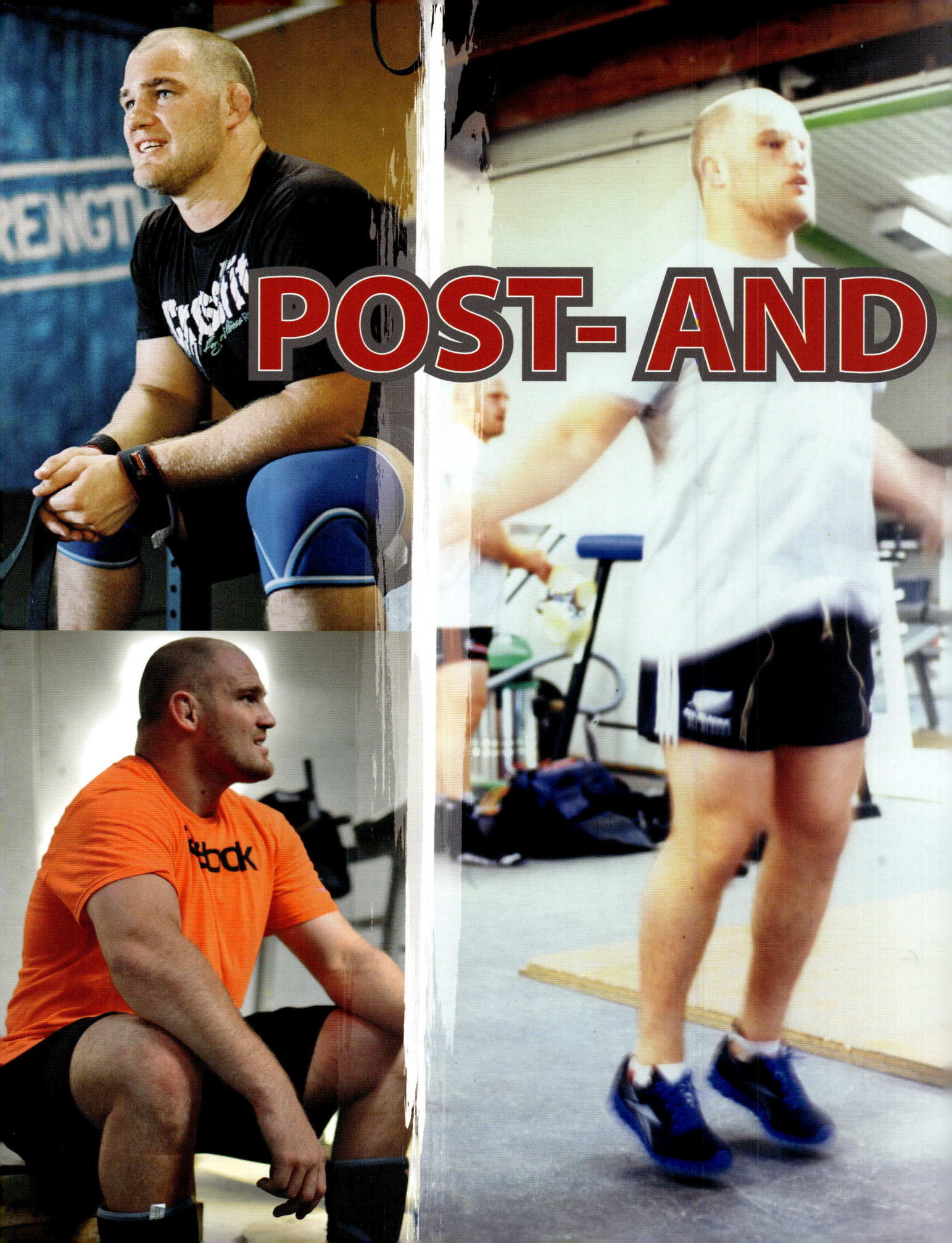

POST- AND

PRE-SEASON TRAINING

Throughout any given year nothing will give you more experience than the in-season game itself, but after the season has finished the greatest opportunities for physical improvement can be found during the off season.

Since rugby union turned professional in 1996 the calendar of a typical rugby player has continued to evolve. Excluding the extensive domestic and international travel, commercial promotions and general outside commitments, having a game scheduled every week requires an athlete to focus on more immediate physical issues outside of getting fitter and stronger.

Recovery, injury prevention, teamwork, strategy, specific skills all tend to dominate most professional athletes' in-season routine. The short time outside of the season is the greatest opportunity for pros to work on weaknesses and develop and strengthen their overall game. Most importantly, this is the best chance to further develop the body and will gradually separate the hard-working from the lazy athletes. At the end of the day, the guy or girl working the hardest will eventually come out on top.

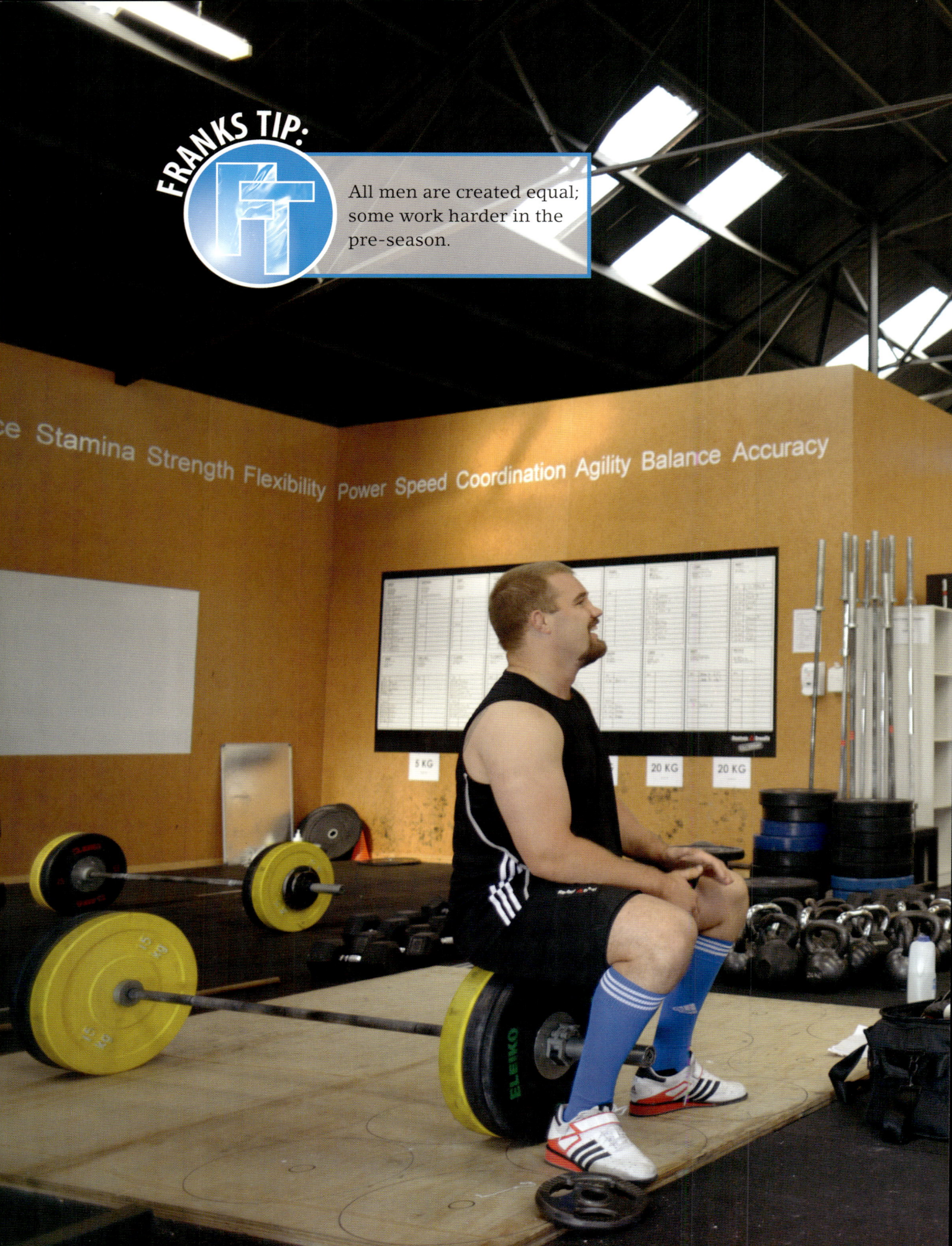

FRANKS TIP:

All men are created equal; some work harder in the pre-season.

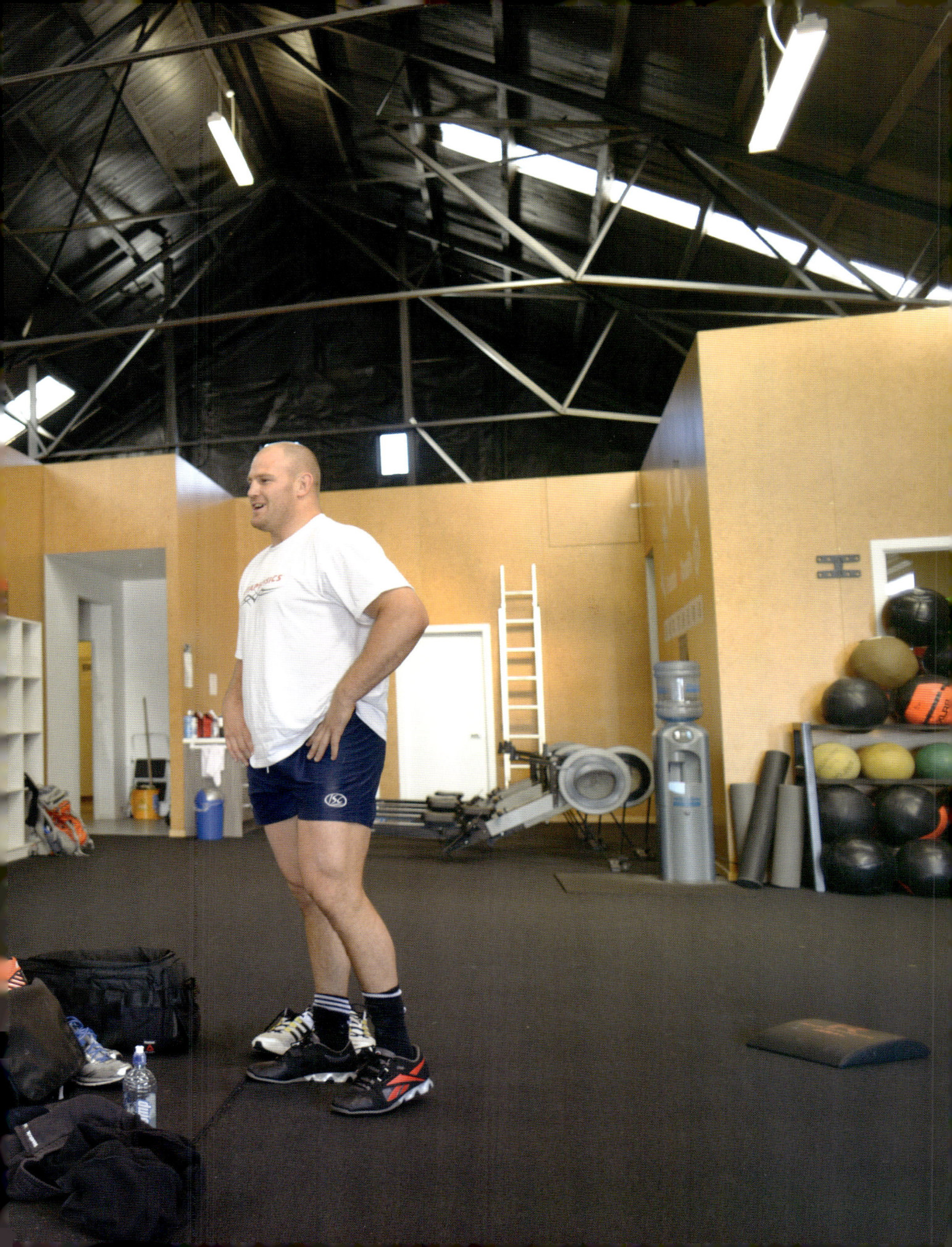

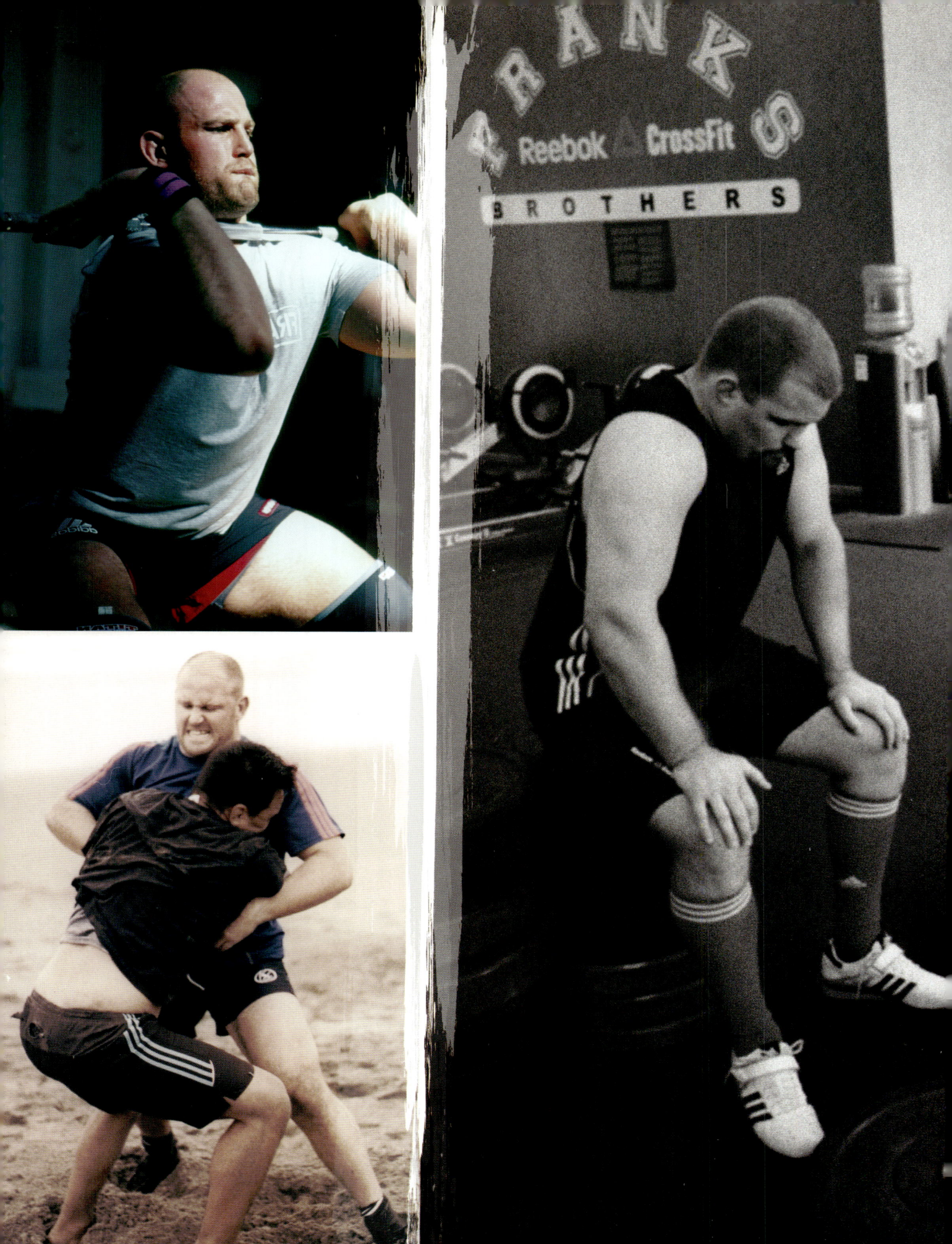

INFLUENCES

Training is hard work.

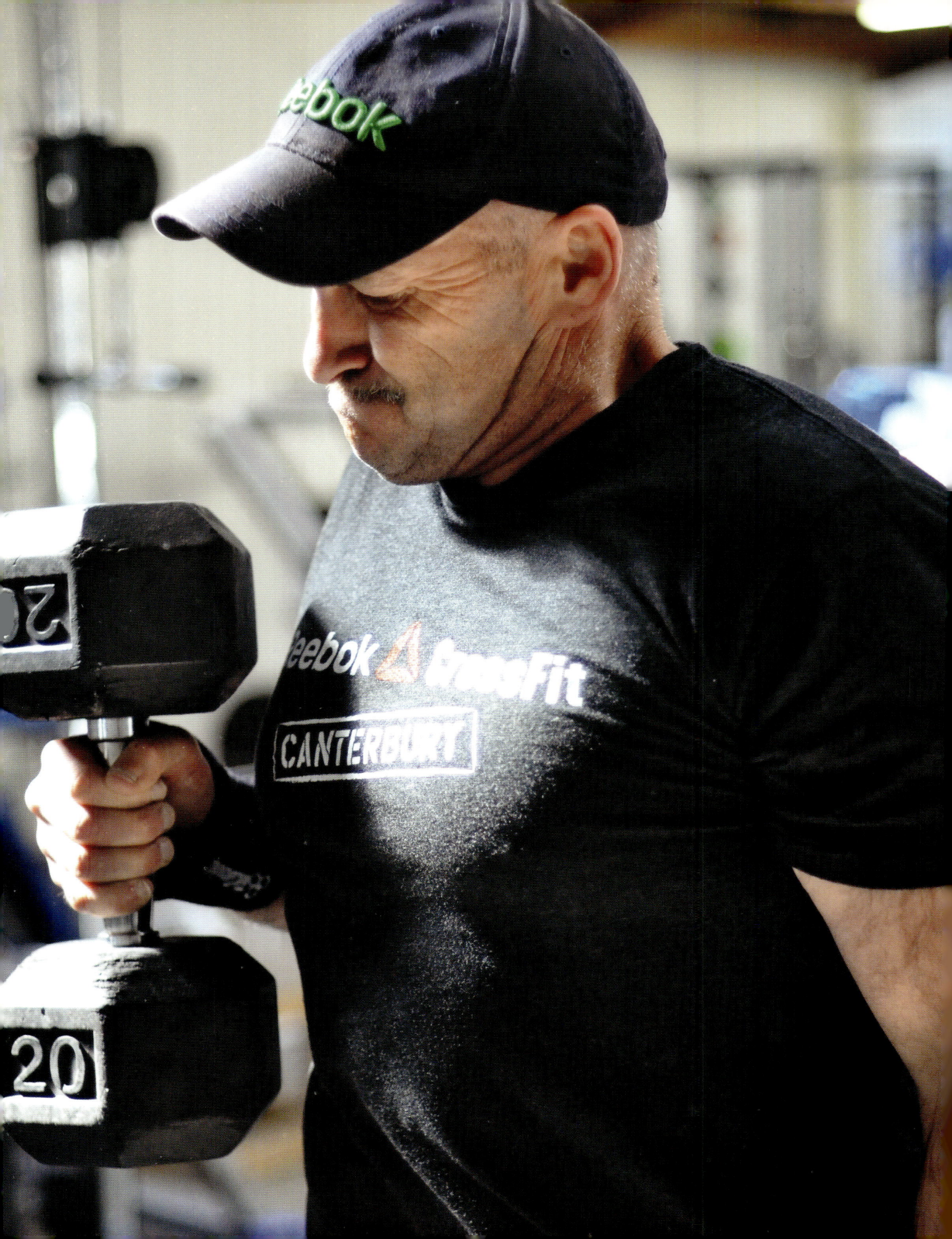

Ken Franks
CrossFit

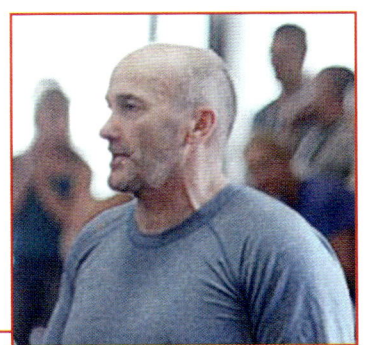

From day one Ken warned his teenage boys that if they each wanted to become professional athletes they would need to make a few difficult sacrifices.

For example, when their friends from school were out chilling at the beach Ben and Owen would need to be running hill sprints or lifting weights. Ken's advice was simple: if you want to get better at something, you need to work hard at it.

While some teenage boys may have rebelled against their father's advice, Ben and Owen committed to the decision to become pro rugby players. Initially, the brothers were average-sized kids. Ken knew a thing or two about exercising but did some extra research and designed a simple plan for the boys to try after school. Owen vividly recalls being 'Dad's guinea pigs' for a few years as a variety of exercises were implemented into their daily exercise program.

While the exercises were important in developing the Franks brothers, what was most important was committing to a training schedule at a young age. By the time Ben's body had matured he had already developed a sustainable training philosophy that both he and Owen continue today.

Over those years Ken has also formally developed his skills as a personal trainer and is currently coaching fulltime at the family-owned Franks Brothers CrossFit gym in Christchurch. Nowadays Ken coaches hundreds of aspiring athletes. His training philosophies continue to evolve and he still works closely with his sons to share successful techniques.

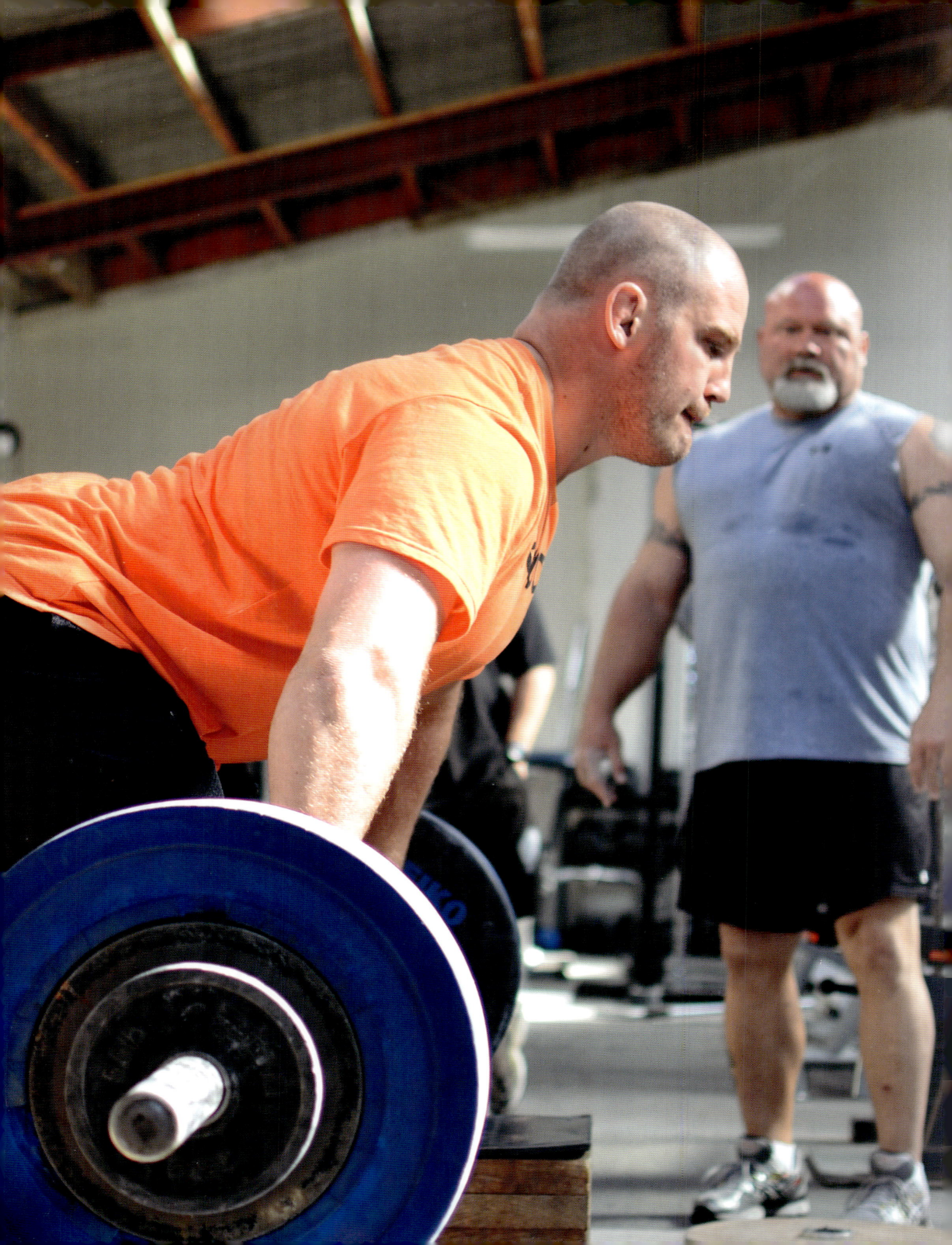

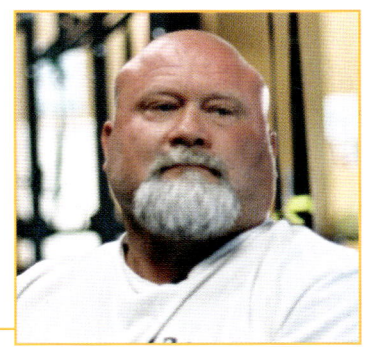

Ed Cosner
Strength and conditioning

American NFL, pro boxing, and NBA are but a few sports that US-based trainer Ed has been involved in.

Building quality explosive athletes is Ed's speciality. His programs are designed to make you stronger and more explosive regardless of your discipline. Ed has his own traditional hard-knocks gym based in the US. During the off season Ben has been known to fly over to the States for extra training with Ed (and other pro US trainers). More recently, however, during the last off season Ben flew Ed to Christchurch city specifically to train together. These training sessions never last longer than an hour but are brutal. In training, a 'Personal Best' or 'PB' is termed when you successfully lift a weight heavier than ever before. Last post-season Ben broke all of his PBs. Ed and Ben would train through the week and take the weekend off to recover and see the local sights.

How you spend your 'holiday time' is up to you, but this ideal training time often separates the good from the great. Check out Ed's training program at the back of the book to see what advice he recommends.

Ed Cosner has played and coached sport professionally for more than 20 years and is world renowned for his work in the strength and conditioning fields. He has a simple philosophy: 'I move beyond the hype and training fads to focus on explosive strength and speed, the foundation of championship performance. My single goal is the creation of champion athletes both on and off the field by using educated and proven scientific principles. By applying expert tests and evaluations and by taking into consideration short and long term goals, I write a training program that is tailor-made to the individual athlete. At that point, drawing on my experience as an athlete, coach and general motivator, I work with the athlete to ensure that gains made in the gym show up in the heat of athletic competition as well as in their everyday lives.' As an aside, Ed has successfully lifted 400 kg on the back squat on a number of occasions.

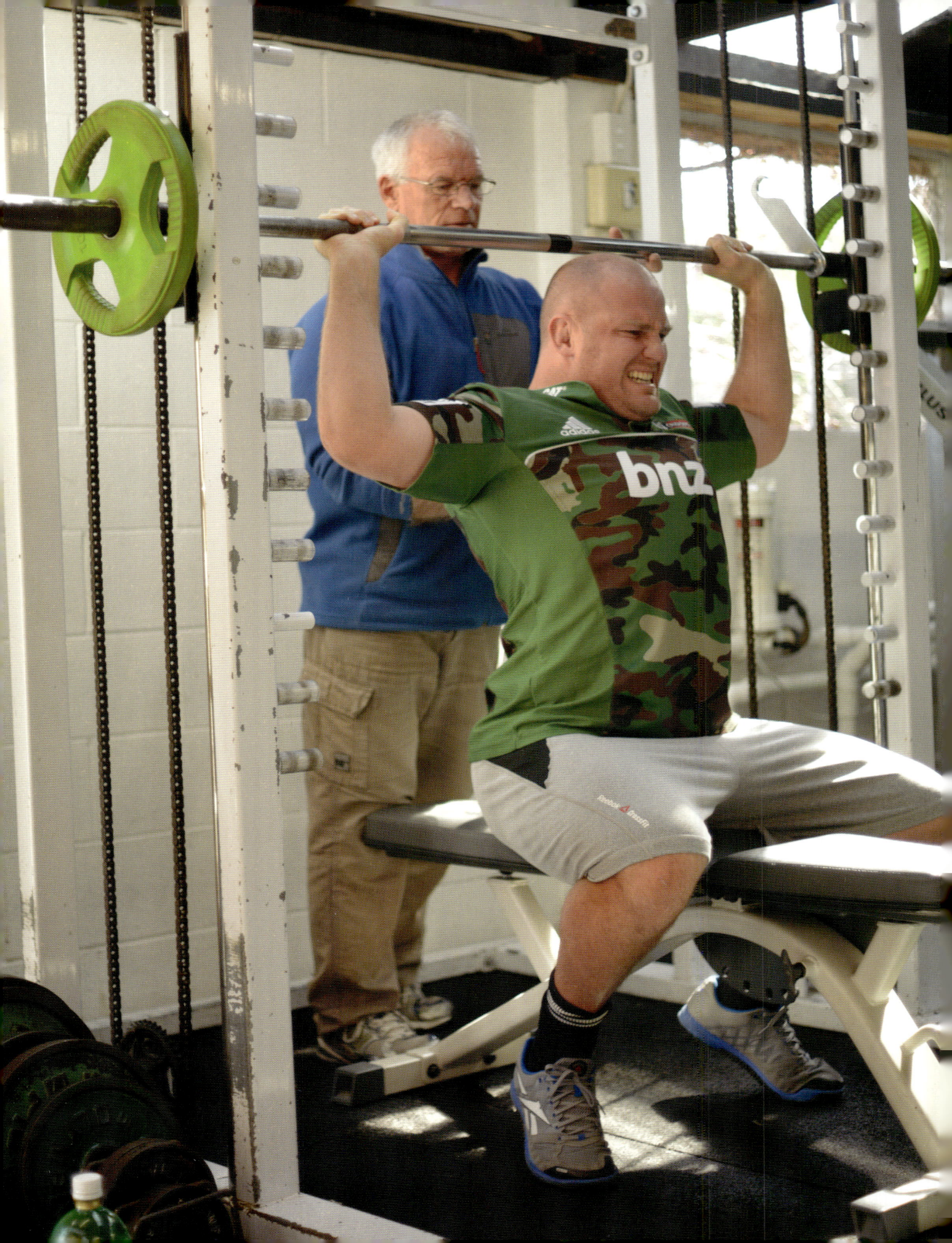

Warren Thin
Bodybuilding

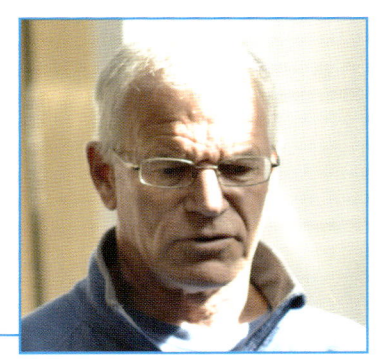

Ben Franks and Warren Thin have been training together since 1997, back when Ben was just 13 years old.

During the 1980s, before Warren was a bodybuilding trainer, he built a solid legacy competing in the Mr New Zealand Bodybuilding Championships. During the 1970s and 1980s bodybuilding was in its prime. The sport was producing wrestlers and Hollywood actors that were quickly becoming household names.

The eight-time Mr New Zealand Bodybuilding Champion learnt a thing or two about developing the body, and through his athlete students Warren continues to grow some of the best muscle around.

Unlike Olympic weightlifting, bodybuilding training targets only a few individual muscles per training session: loading the muscle up until it fails repetitively, and then allowing it to rest and grow. Obviously, there is a little more to growing muscle than that. Good-quality food, circulation, and rest after training all contribute to development. The training session itself consists of short, sharp bursts so that even though you are only working a few muscles at a time, by the end your heart rate and breathing are at maximum. Bodybuilders load the muscle up so that only 8 to 12 relations are possible from whichever muscle group is being worked.

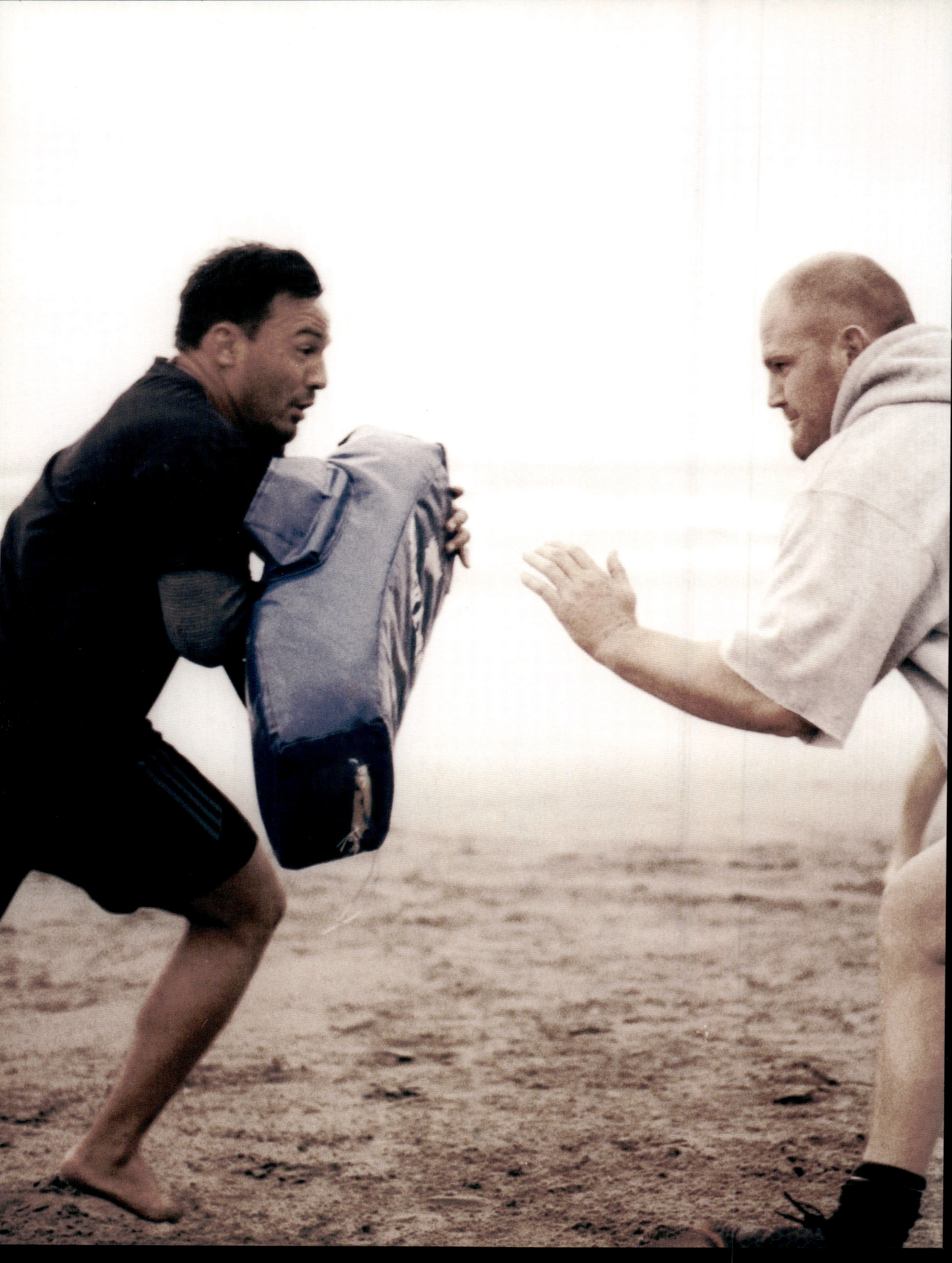

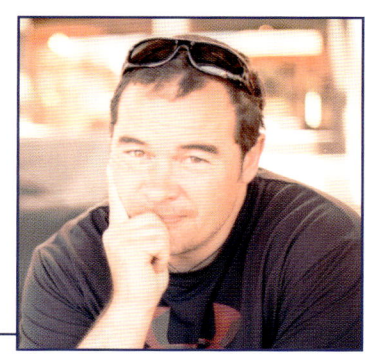

Scott Hansen
Rugby training

While running shuttles and lifting weights will help with your overall condition, nothing will help you on your journey to improve at your sport more than the sport itself.

Ben and Owen Franks have been students of rugby union from a young age and have received a great education on the intricacies of the game from a variety of coaches – none more than the advice from Canterbury-based coach/trainer Scott Hansen.

During the off season there is a two-month window where Scott enjoys putting the brothers through their paces. After a heavy session in the gym Scott recommends balancing the training day with either some hand–eye coordination, fast explosive movements, or technique drills.

It is not uncommon to find Ben and Owen and some energetic young hopefuls lined up at the beach during the early hours of the morning practising tackle techniques with the pads or using each other as tackle dummies.

Scott Hansen is a former Crusaders and Canterbury halfback. He is currently manager of the Linwood Rugby Club with special responsibility for pre-season skills and drills with the club. He has worked with Ben and Owen for six years.

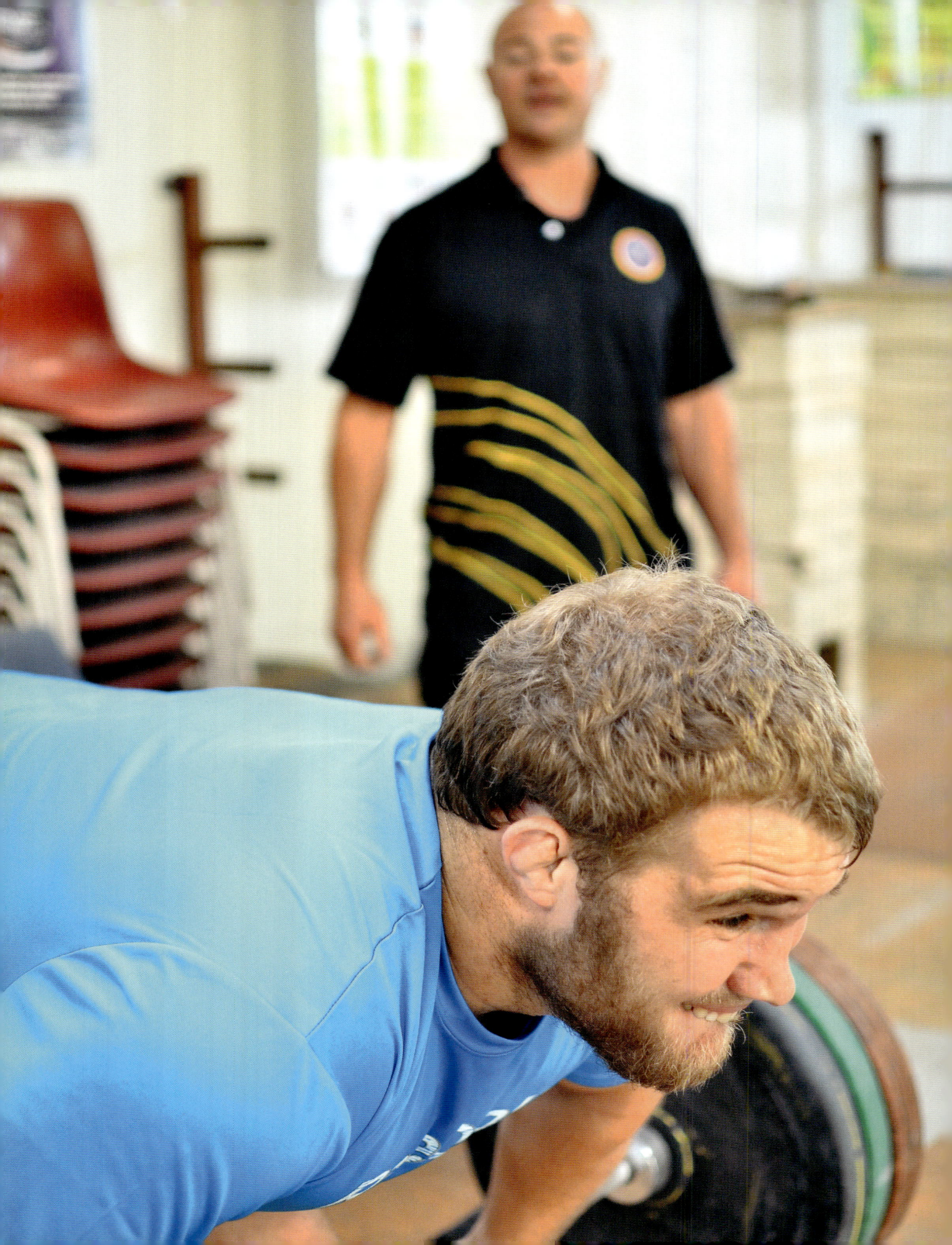

Lee Attrill
Olympic lifting coach

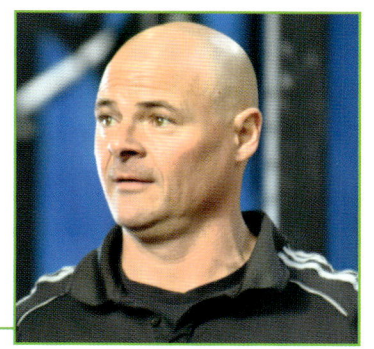

For a 13th birthday present Ken Franks signed each of his boys up to the local Olympic lifting club.

By then the pair had made a mental commitment to become professional rugby players, but back then many people did not believe that the Franks brothers possessed enough size to become world-class rugby players – let alone World Cup-winning All Blacks.

Owen, for example, would generally not make local school-grade selection for the 1st, or sometimes 2nd, rugby teams. But Ken would remain positive. Like many great athletes who did not get selected at a young age, this provided fuel and motivation to establish a solid training routine that ultimately developed the habits required in building a more competitive body. Lee Attrill, through Olympic lifting, played a huge role in that development.

Over the last 15 years Lee Attrill has continued to build a strong base for the Franks brothers through Olympic lifting. The classic 'clean' is one of the most common exercises found in the Franks routine. Lee will tell you this movement is the basis of Ben and Owen's strength and power. The 'clean' is a fundamental Olympic movement and is one of the most explosive exercises for the physical body. Posture and speed is key. Watching Ben and Owen knock out 5 sets of 3 reps makes the movement look too easy.

Lee Attrill represented New Zealand in Olympic weightlifting at the 1994 Commonwealth Games in Victoria, Canada. These days he is an Olympic weightlifting and strength coach. Lee's best competition snatch was 140 kg, while his best clean and jerk was 182.5 kg.

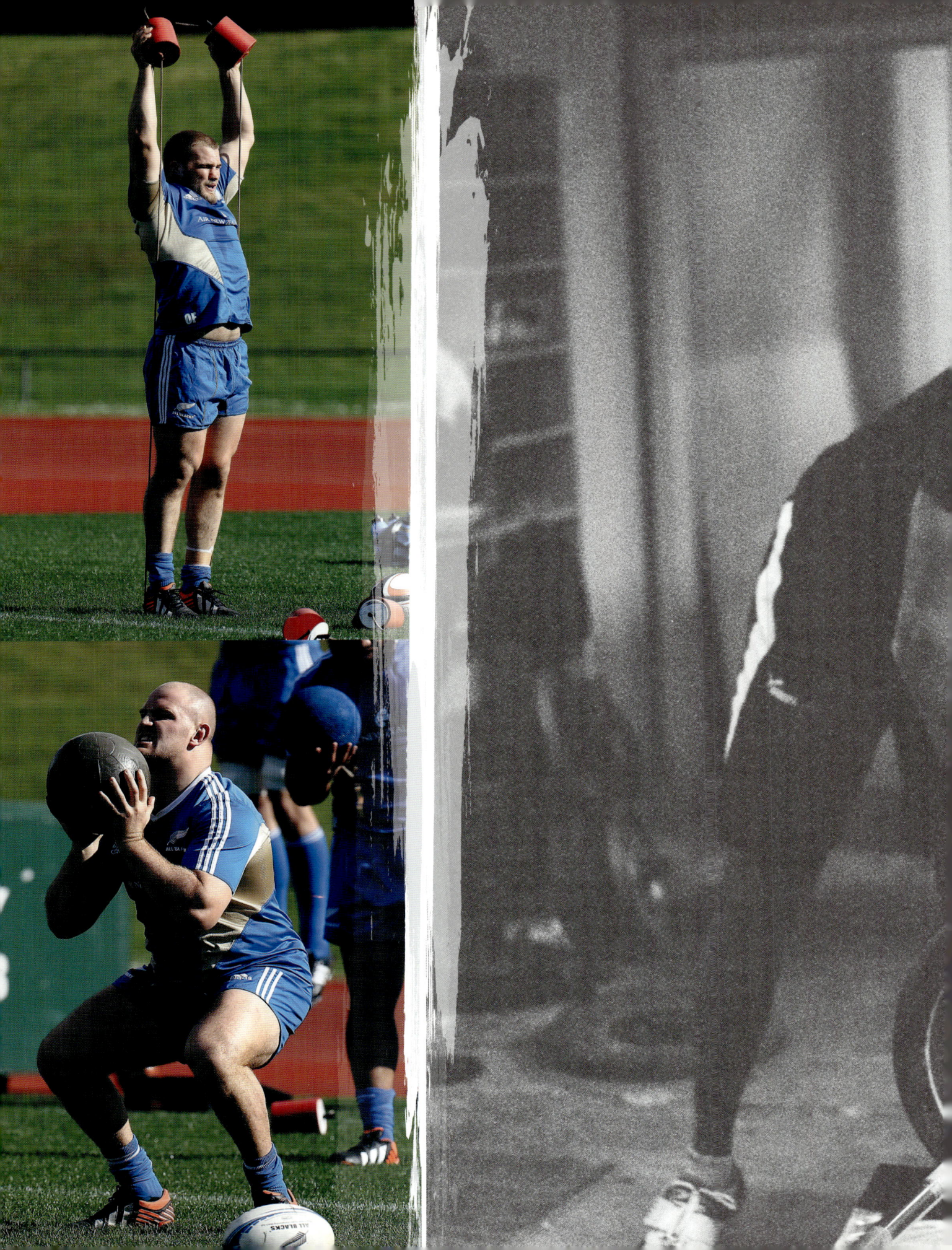

EQUIPMENT

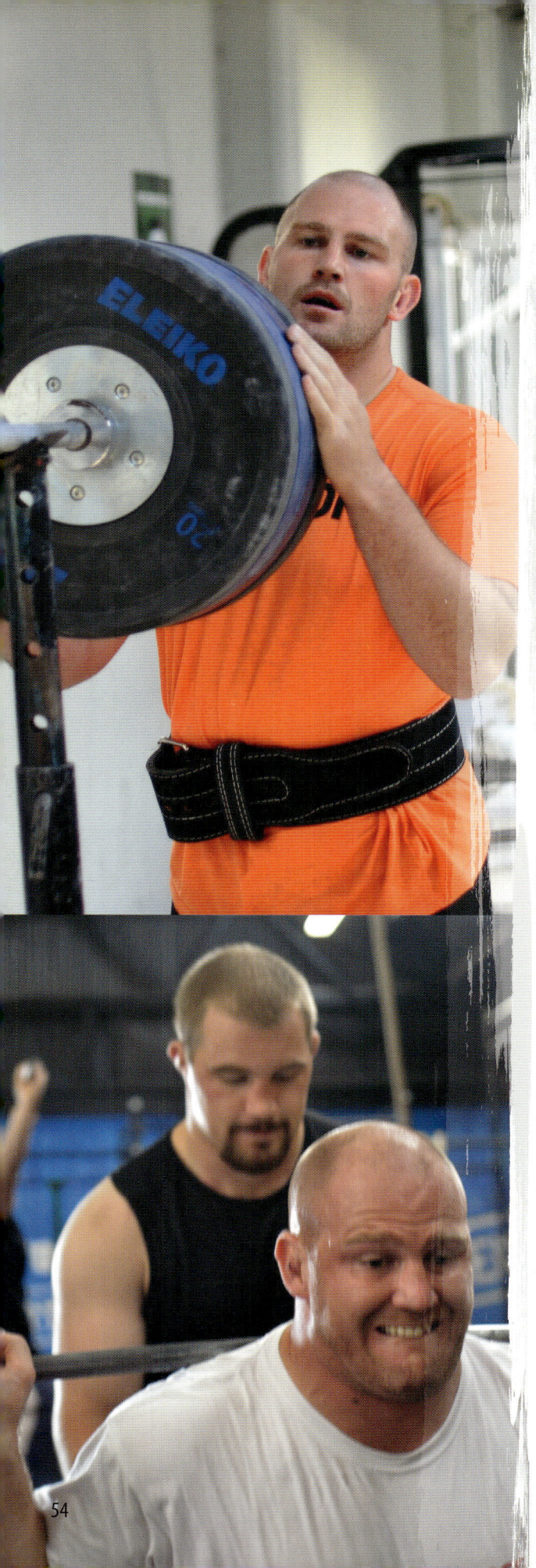

Weights

If you are training at a public gym, all you need is a towel and a drink bottle. If, however, you are training from home the main piece of equipment you will need is a bar and some plates. Initially, just using the bar without any extra weight is a good way to start while learning the correct movements and improving on overall technique. If you continue to train at a home gym, investing in pairs of 5 kg and 10 kg plates every so often will become a recurring theme as you get stronger.

A bench-press frame is a helpful tool, but not mandatory. If you don't have access to a bench, or you want to be like the Franks CrossFit gym, just use the floor.

An exercise as basic as the front squat (see page 95) still requires a strict centred movement. As you slowly get stronger over time you will need to invest in more weight to add on.

Drink bottle

Drinking plenty of water is the most important dietary habit an athlete must develop. Dehydration will dramatically lower the intensity of your exercise. Drink a glass of water when you wake up. Better yet, keep a drink bottle by your bed. If you've had a hard day training it is not unusual to wake up in the middle of the night thirsty. Your body is made up of 70 per cent water and doesn't enjoy anything less than that. If during training your mouth is dry and after training you find your muscles cramping, chances are you haven't consumed enough water before and after the session.

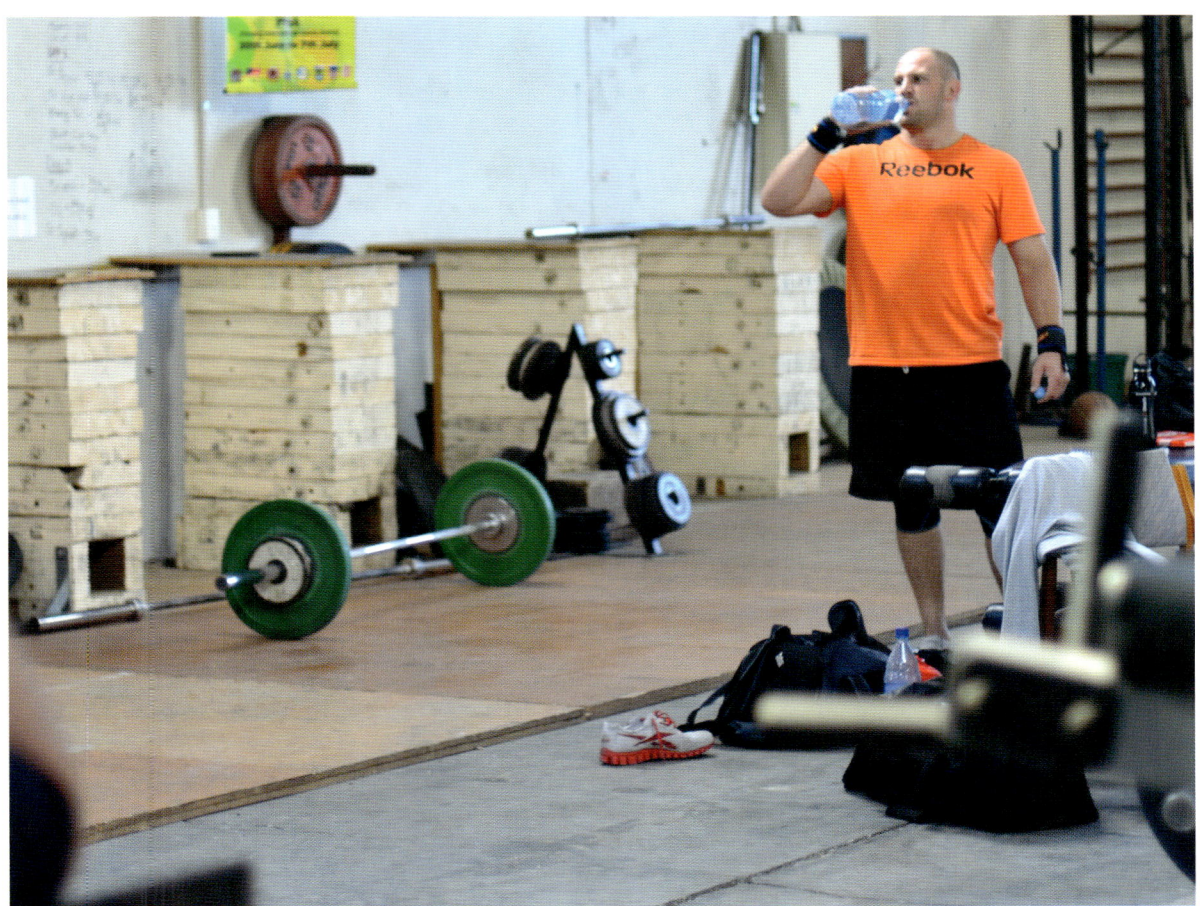

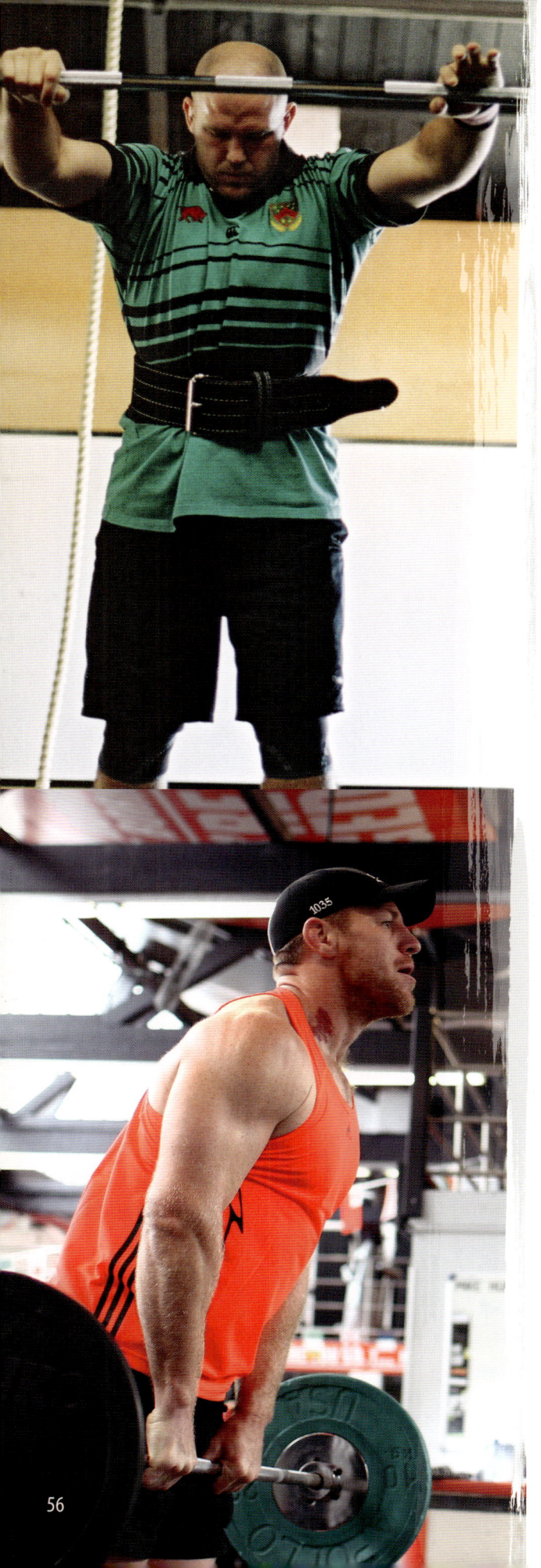

Clothing

In most cases professional athletes like Ben and Owen will receive an annual crate full of sponsors' products to wear for the season, as well as a budget to spend on any other equipment or clothing they need from the catalogue. Then, when training with the Crusaders or the All Blacks, the team will be advised what uniform and colours to wear, and in the backline's case, causing panic about what coloured shoes to match.

You, however, can wear whatever you are comfortable with. Synthetic fabrics tend to hold less sweat – although you will get more head nods and hat tips from the Franks if you are sporting a heavy cotton Canterbury Linwood rugby jersey. Gym buff and close friend Brad Thorn is well known by teammates for religiously wearing a tight singlet while working out. But be warned. Gym conservatives may have a thing or two to say about 'hot-dogging in the gym' which may rule out the matching adidas jumpsuit with cut-off sleeves until you have earned the legendary status of Brad or at least until you end up on the set of a Les Mills commercial.

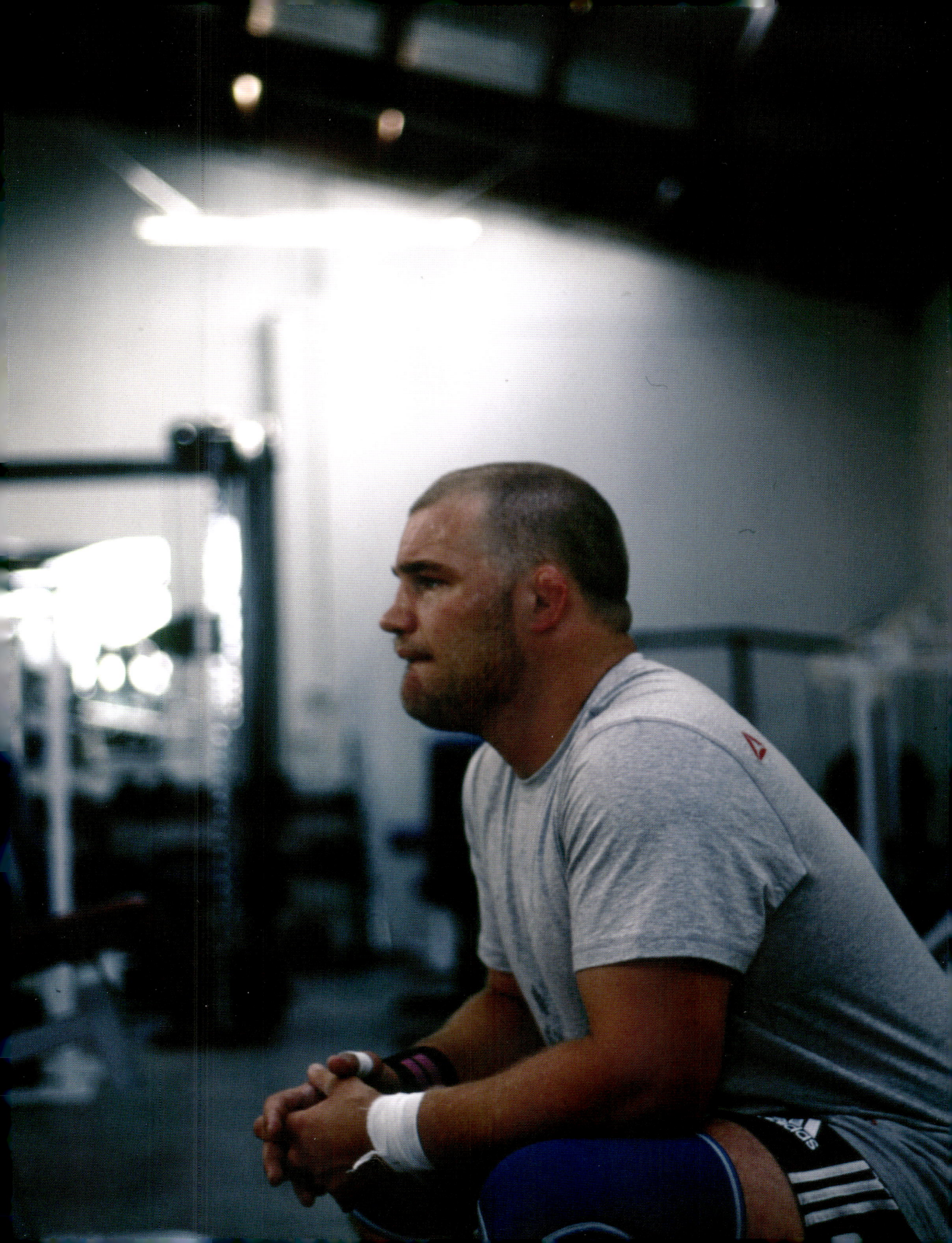

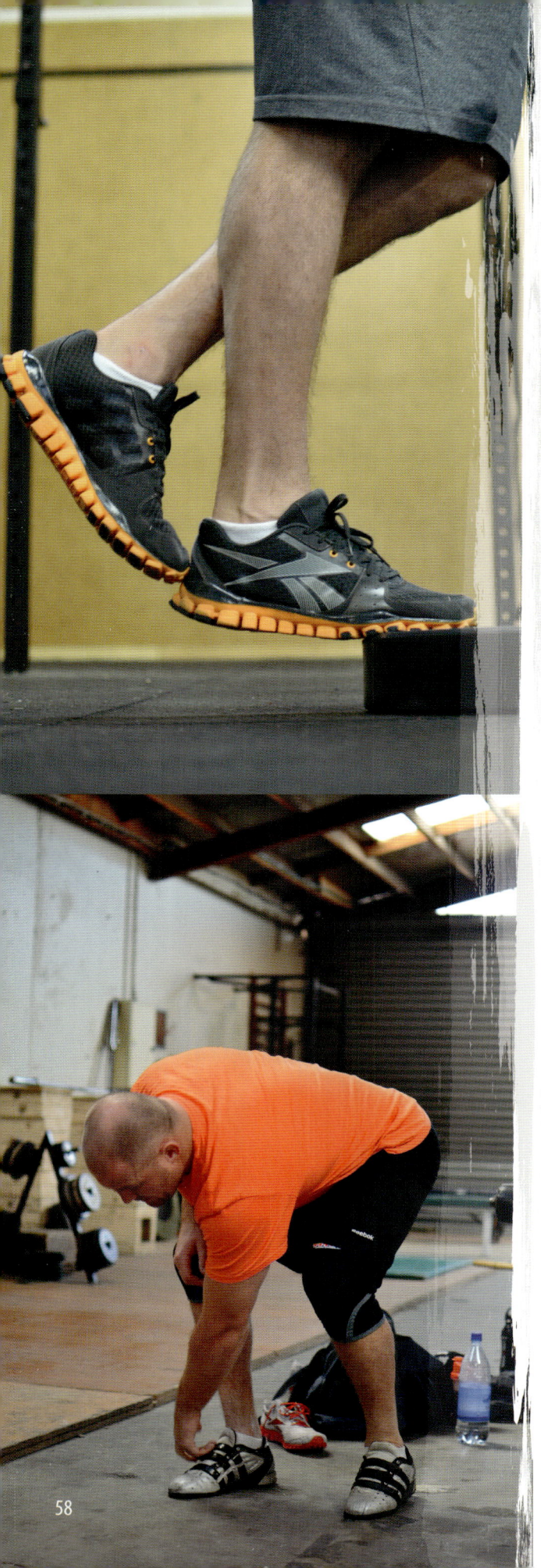

Shoes

Regardless whether you are just starting out with training or have been working out for some time, your best option regarding footwear is to make an appointment with your local podiatrist. Specialists will advocate that your body's entire posture starts at your feet. Got a problem with your neck? It could be all due to the pronation or supination (roll or rotation) of your feet. Inspect the sole of your favourite shoes and see if the wear is even across the sole. If your shoe looks to be collapsing in, or out, take it with you to your local podiatrist.

If you are lucky enough to have a 'neutral' foot, you can safely train in any flat neutral shoe. Ideally, you would have an array of shoes for every purpose: a spongy running shoe for running, a wooden-heeled Olympic lifting shoe for heavy lifting, and a sprigged boot for grass field training. However, if you are a young lad with no budget, the Chuck Taylors in the corner of your room might have to do for the moment. And if you are a Rocky movie fan then that is probably all you will train in.

However, in short, weightlifting shoes are the perfect investment for Olympic weightlifting, running shoes are perfect for running, but neither shoe will be ideal for cross-training. Weightlifting shoes have a solid wooden heel while running shoes are not designed to support large amounts of extra weight.

Training log

One of the best ways to stay motivated throughout training is to see progress. Keeping a record of your progress is the habit of every serious professional. Over time you can see how your body is developing in reaction to your training and track the development of its limits. Head the log with the date, followed by the exercises you performed, and the weight and number of repetitions. Keep track of your personal bests, especially during the off season, so you can then strive hard to regularly beat them without having to worry about being fresh for the next club match.

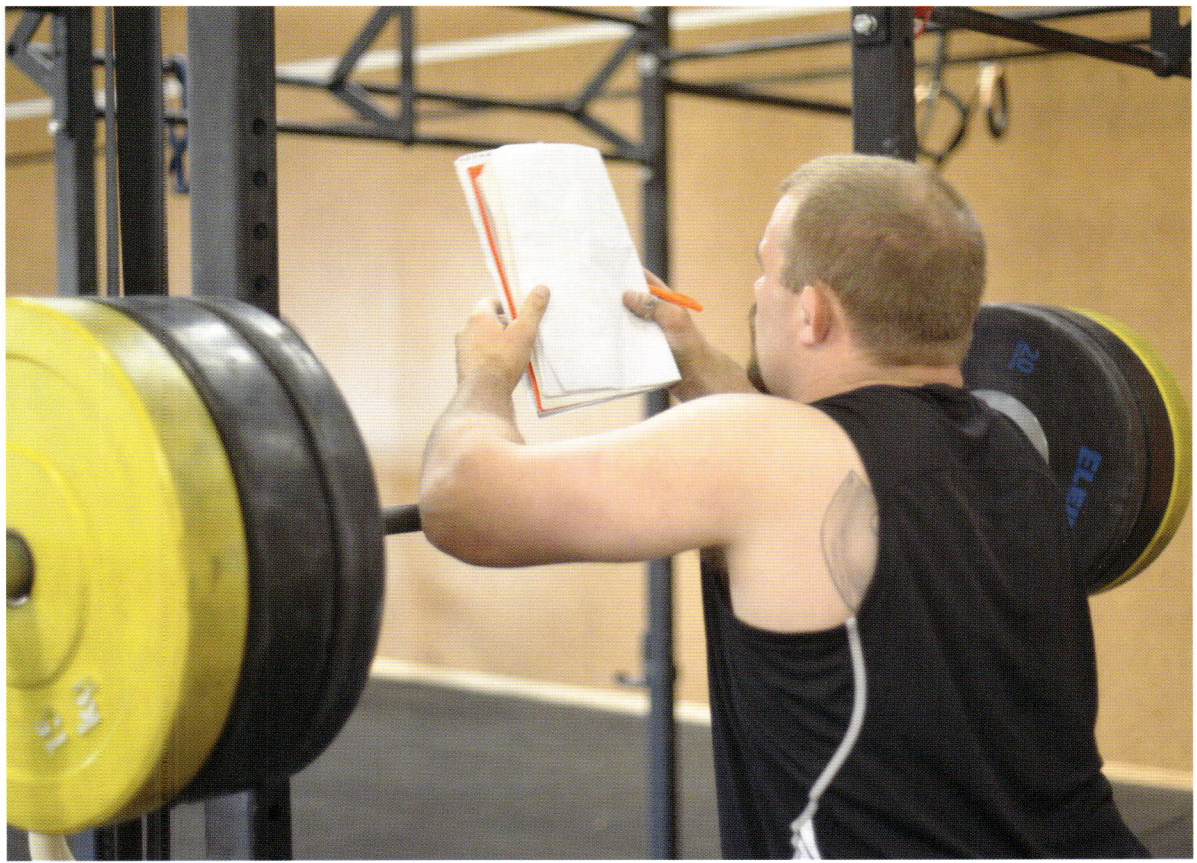

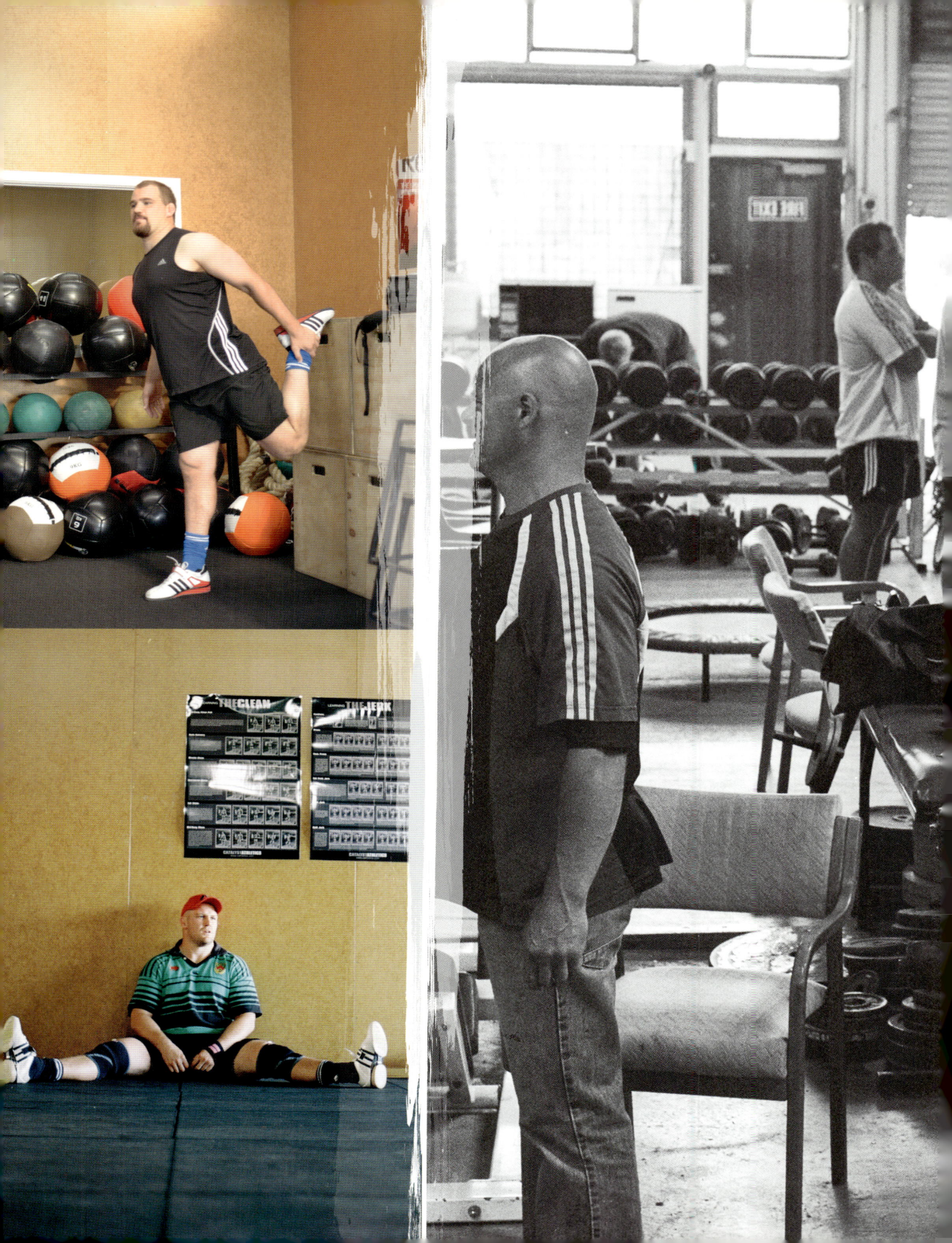

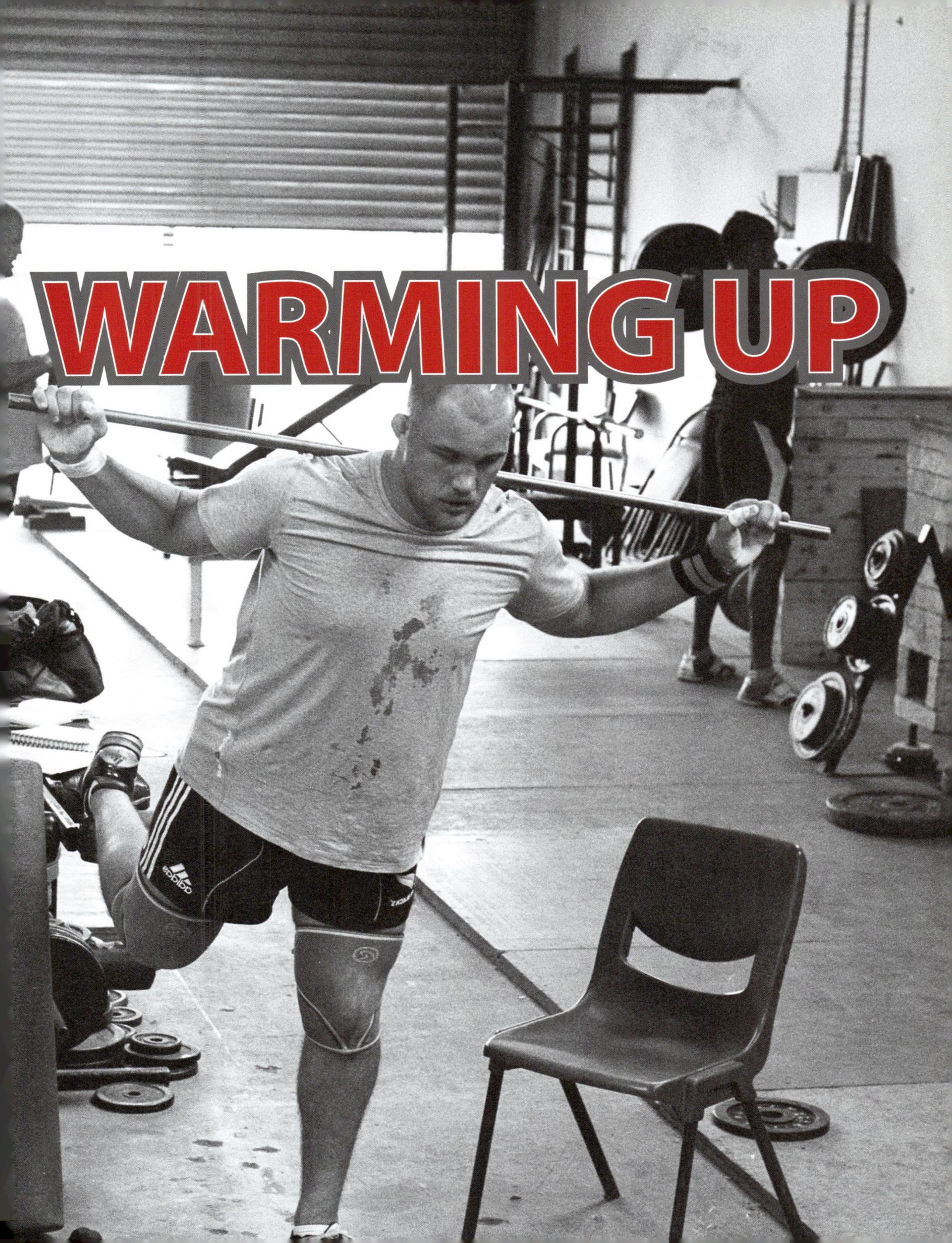

WARMING UP

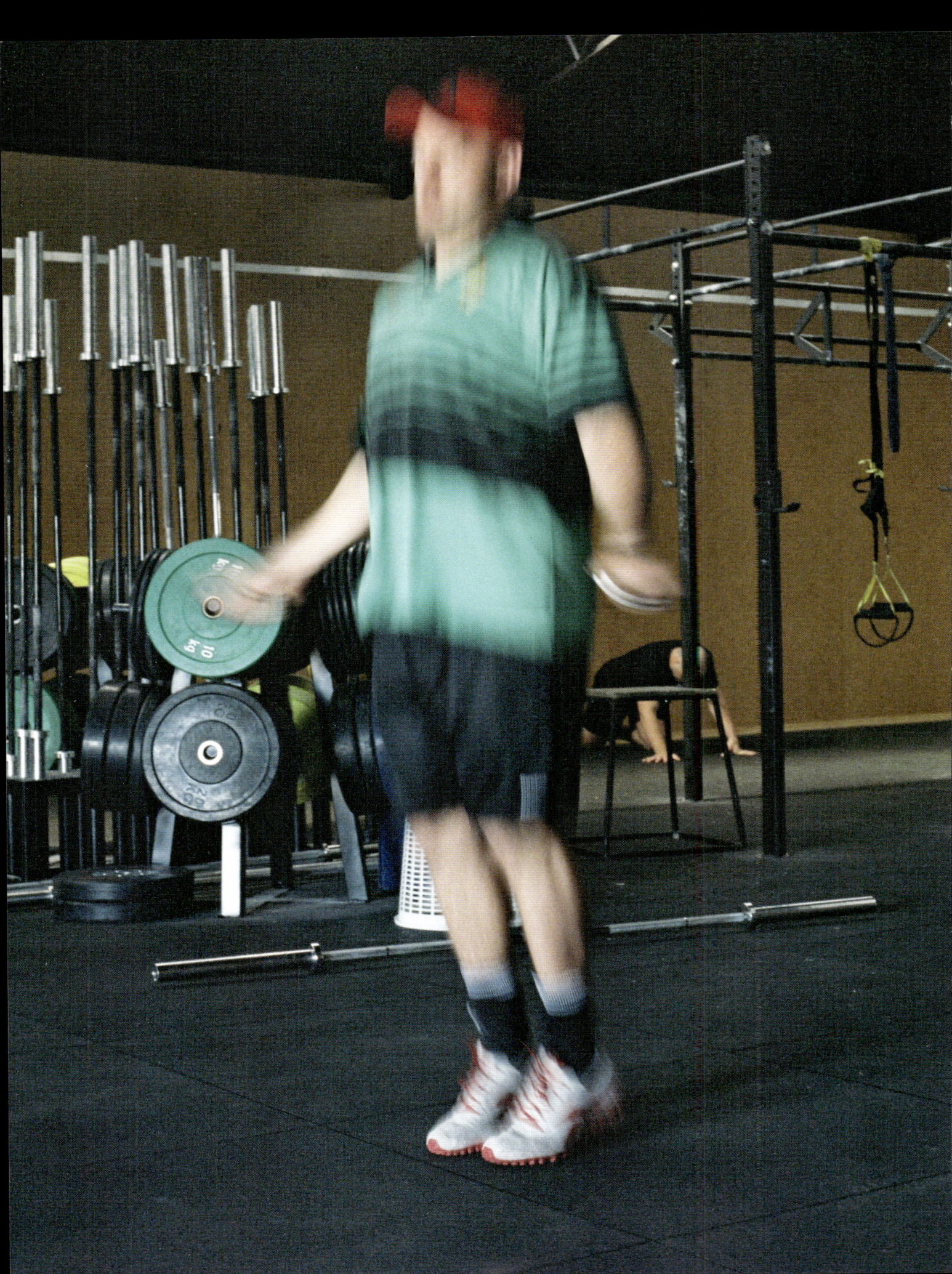

The muscles in your body need to be slowly warmed up then stretched out and taken through their range of motion in order to assure no sprains or tears. The older your body gets, the more important it is to have a warm-up and warm-down routine.

Skipping for 5 to 10 minutes or going for a 1 km jog is a classic way to get a light sweat going but be sure to mix it up. Ten push-ups, sit-ups, and pull-ups would easily break a sweat too. Boxers skip for 10 minutes non-stop. Any which way, have some fun with it. Be sure to stay relaxed and remember that this is a good chance to develop a routine to get focused on the tasks at hand.

Next is stretching. It is considered good practice to stand up tall, open your posture up and lightly stretch the major muscles in your body. Taking your body through its range of motion will help ready the muscles and joints as well as give you a better chance to avoid injury. Take nice big breaths and, starting with your legs up to your neck, hold as many different stretch positions for around 10 seconds each. Holding for longer is better following the training session, after the body has been at full temperature. Stretching is covered in the 'Recovery' section (see page 129).

Once you feel that your body is warm, stretched and ready to go, you can move on to the main event, putting a full effort into your game, match, or training session.

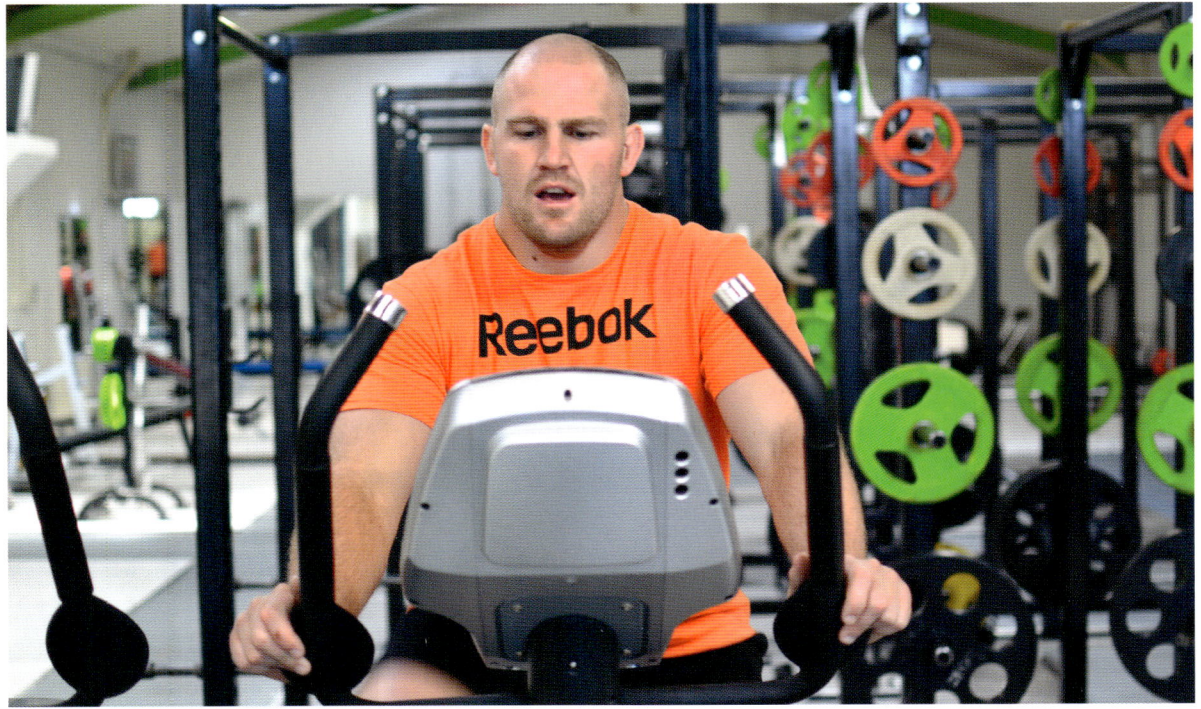

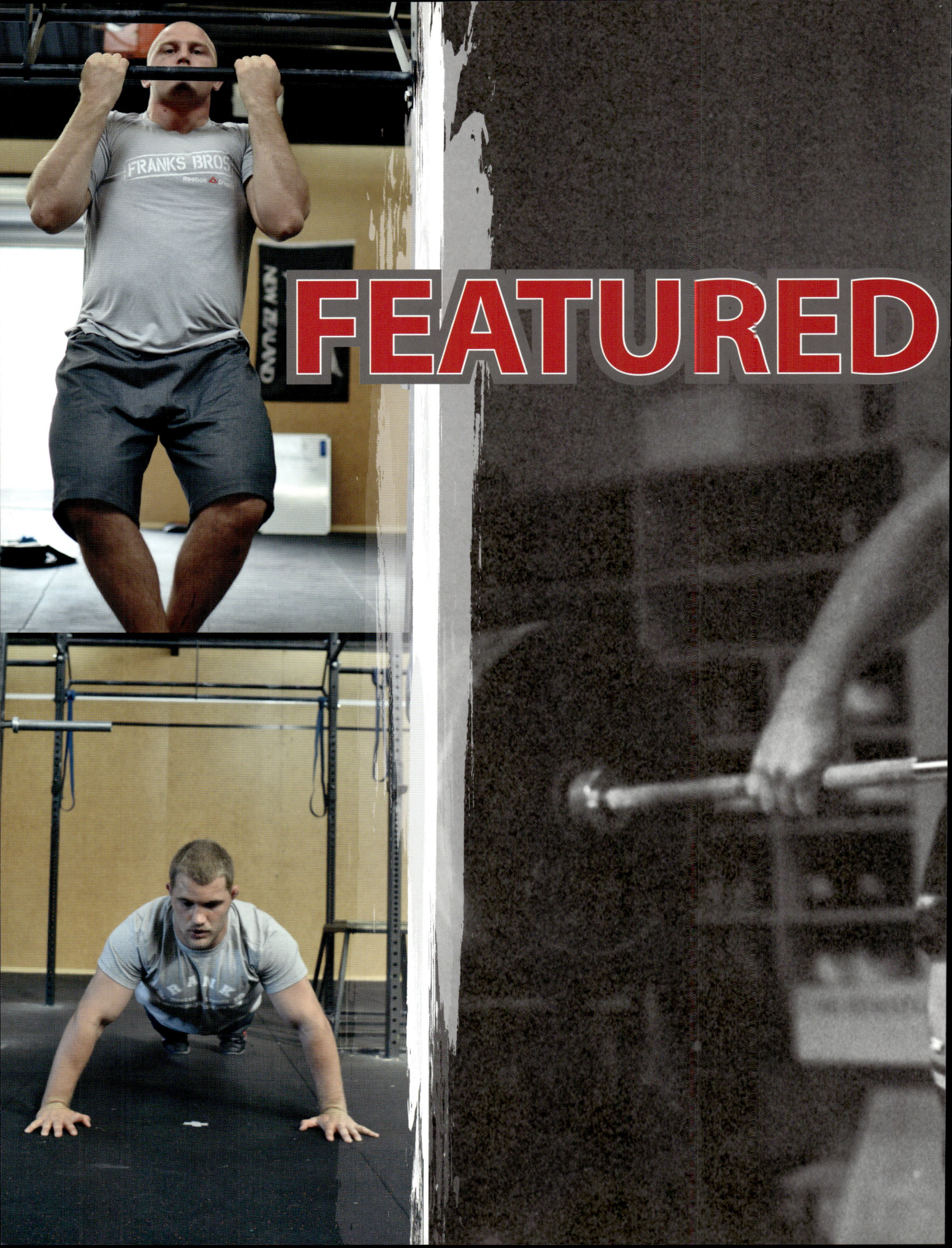

FEATURED

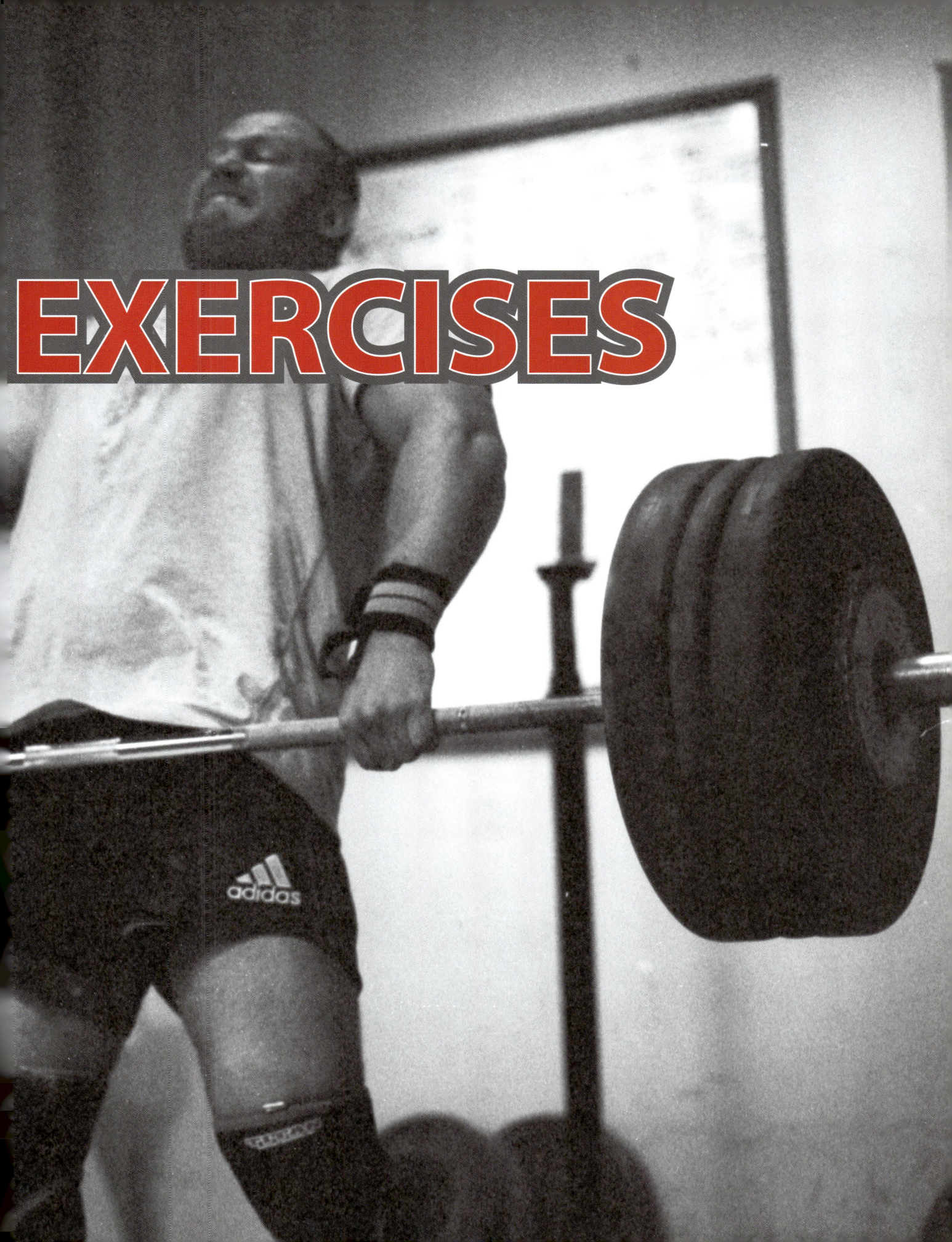

EXERCISES

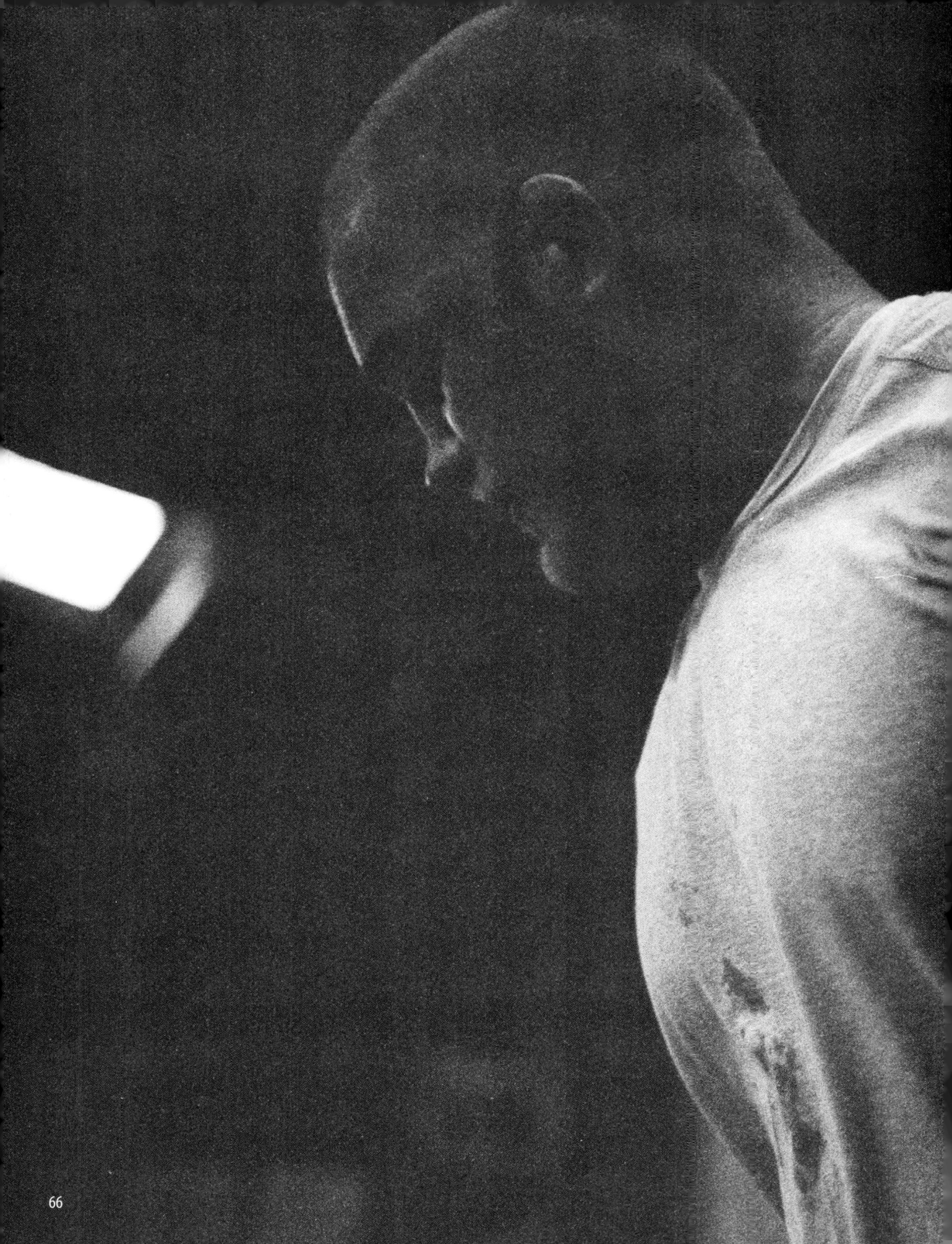

BODYWEIGHT EXERCISES

(featured in order of Bodyweight Circuit #1)

Gravity plus the weight of your body offer more than enough resistance for a beginner. Taking your body through each of the following movements, over time, will provide a good solid base before advancing to lifting extra weights. These movements also act as a recommended warm-up before lifting heavier weights.

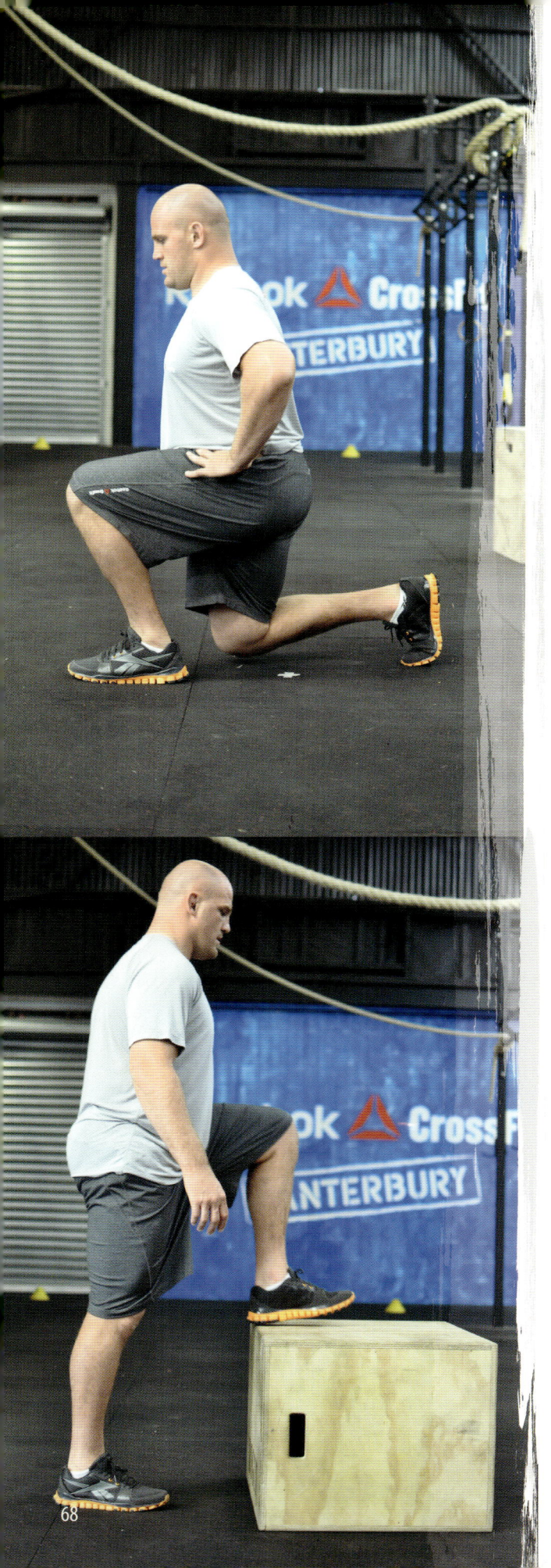

CORE EXERCISES

Your arms and legs are connected together and coordinated by your core. Consider the important fact that if your core isn't strong, your limbs have no solid base to operate from and will ultimately weaken performance. The core muscles featured around your waist and stomach are very important to keep strong. Core muscles connect your arms and legs, providing the fundamental strength to keep your body steady.

Generally speaking, when a rookie athlete is first contracted to a professional sports team, core strength is the very first weakness trainers will address. Close friend, team-mate and gym buff Brad Thorn is renowned for his gut-busting core workouts. Brad prides himself on executing over 200 various core repetitions accumulated between every set of his workout.

An easy way to test your own core strength is to take the 'plank' position on the floor, weight on elbows and toes, and see how long you can hold a flat position. Three minutes is a good time, but if you can't hold for two minutes then you really need to get to work. A full book in itself could be written on the various ways to help develop better strength and endurance in the core muscle groups, but for now just stick to the basics.

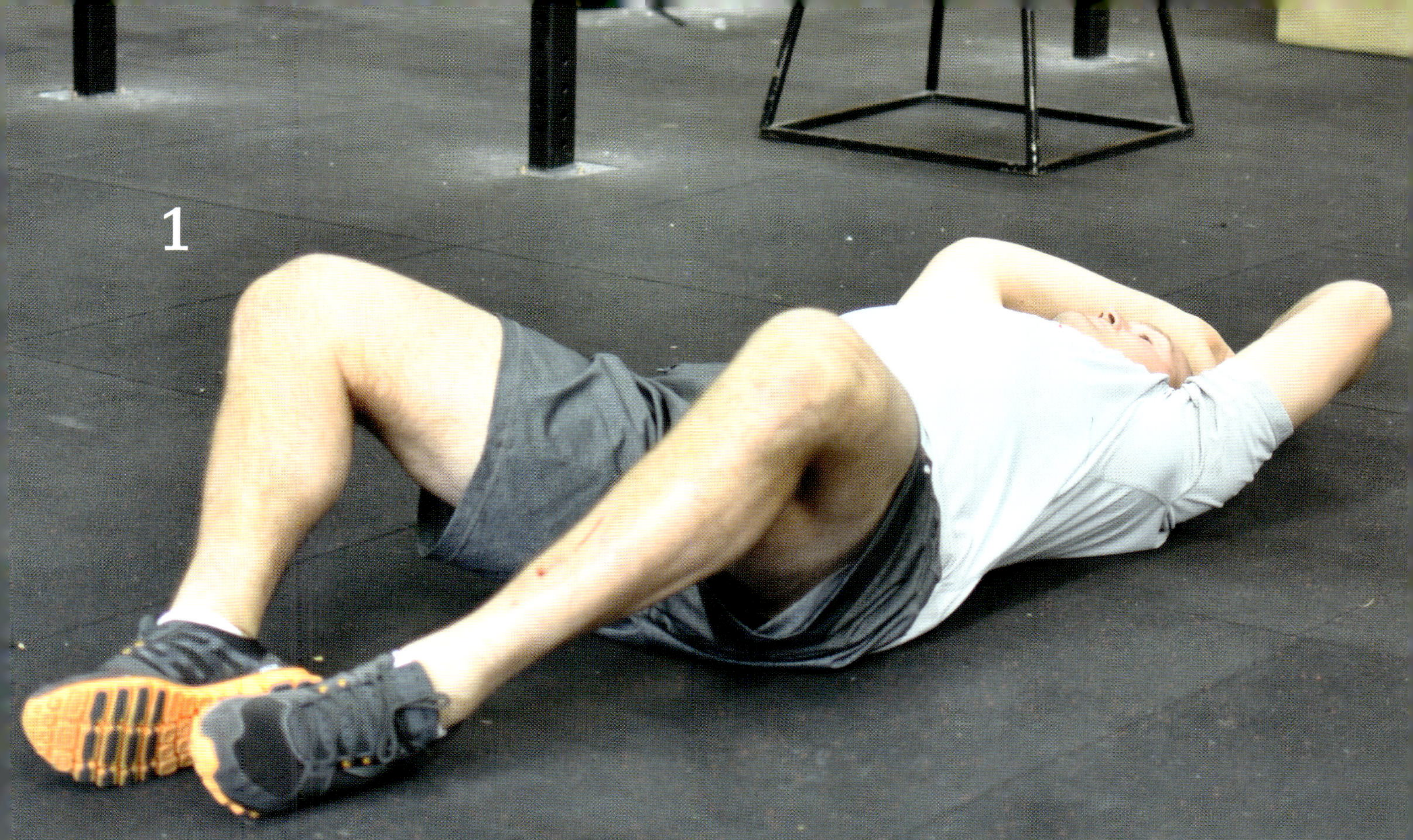

1

Sit-ups

The mainstay of core workouts is sit-ups. Isolate the core muscles simply by placing the soles of the feet together and hands touching. Having your feet opposing each other will make the exercise harder but will provide better long-term gains. Simply sit up and touch your toes and then repeat. Move at a controlled speed. At first see how many you can do in a row and improve from there.

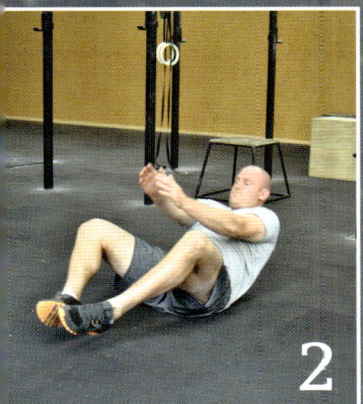

2

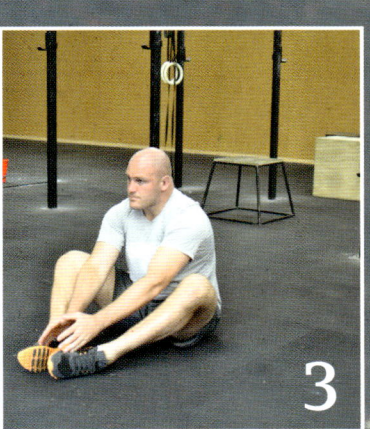

3

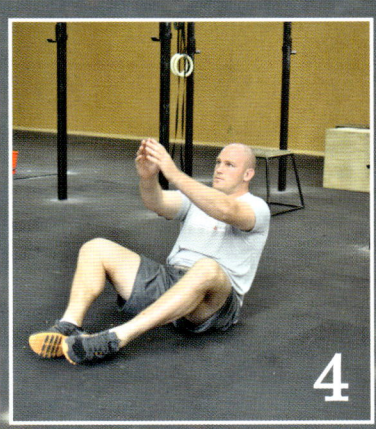

4

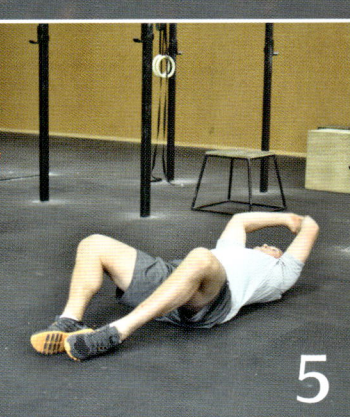

5

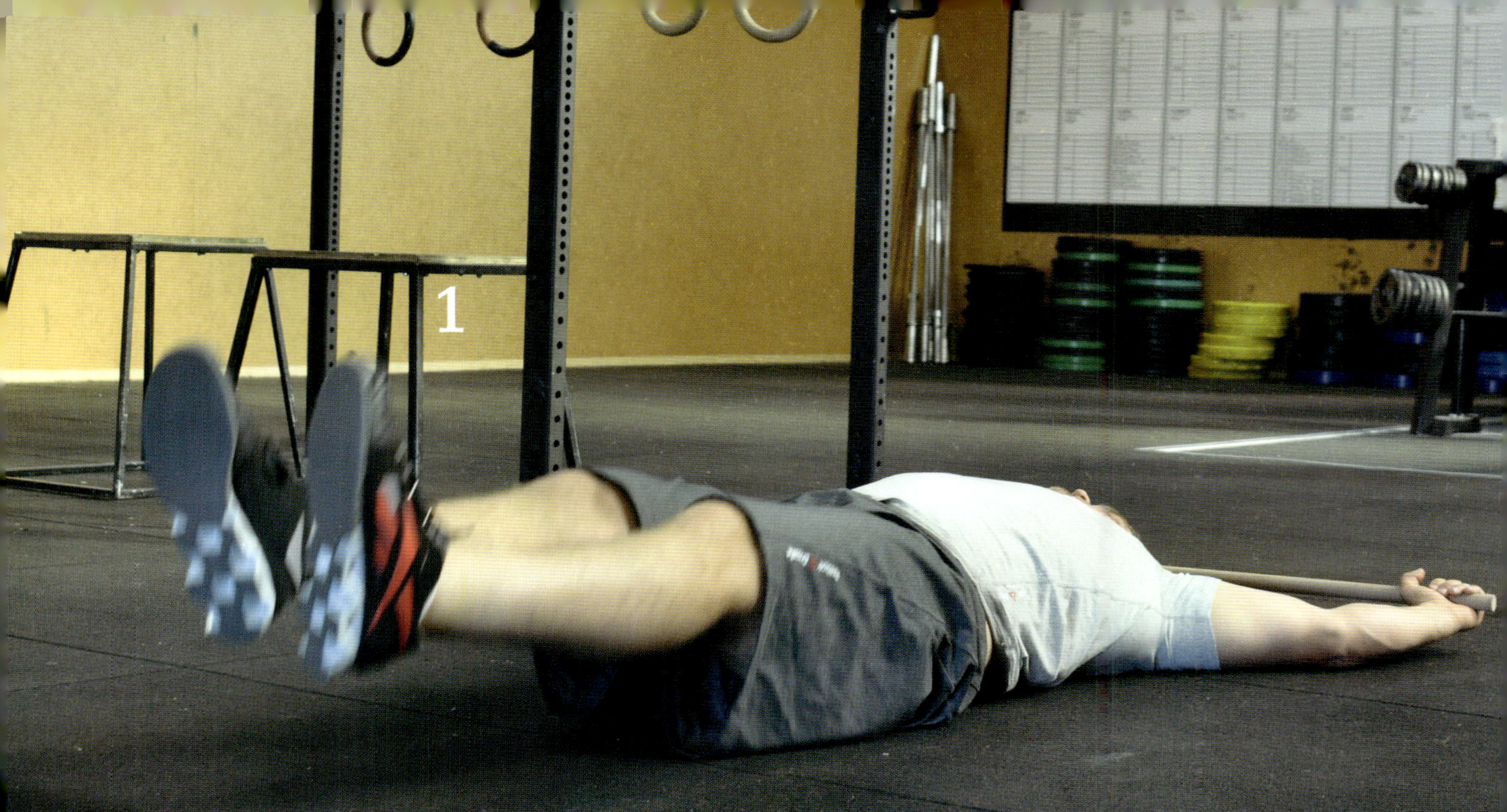

Leg raisers

The leg raiser exercise is a great building block for strengthening the lower abdominal and back muscles. Keep your legs straight while lying on the ground. Either hold a stick/bar above your head, or simply tuck your hands under your backside while lifting the legs up and down. Note how many you can do in a row with a minute's break, finishing 3 sets, and then work on improving that number.

BEGINNERS: 3 sets of 12 reps — with 1 minute break between sets.

INTERMEDIATE: 3 sets of 20 — with 30 seconds break between sets.

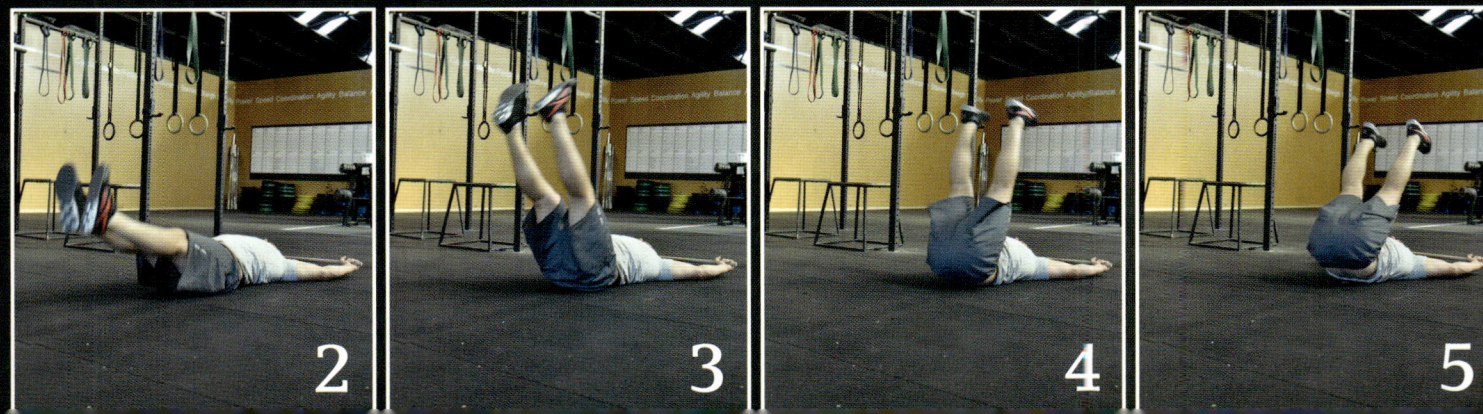

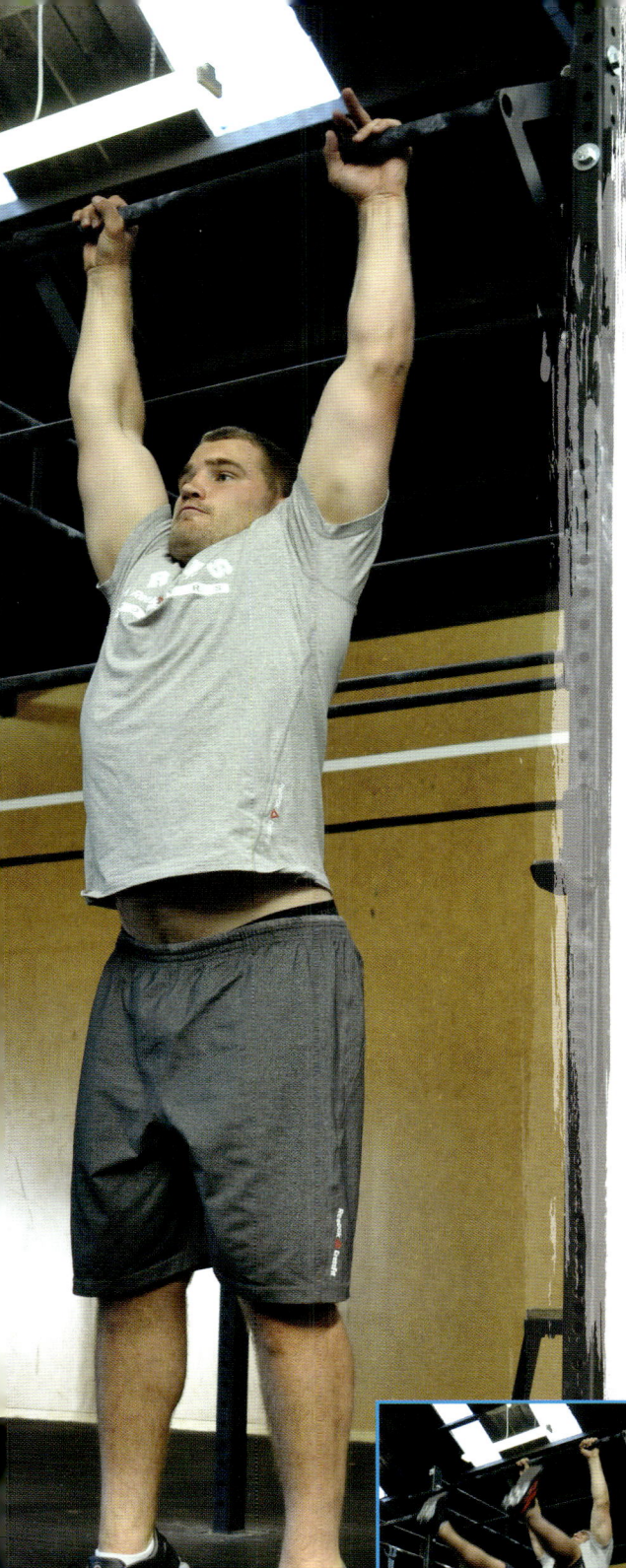

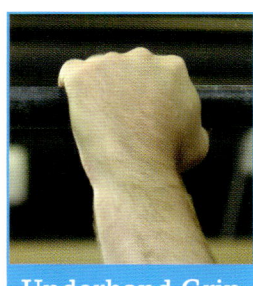
Underhand Grip

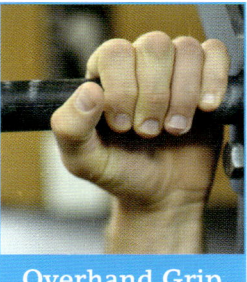
Overhand Grip

Toes to bar

The advanced progression of leg raisers involves more gravity against the legs by hanging from a bar. Using a wide over- or underhand grip (see above), start and finish in a relaxed hanging position. Swiftly engage your lower abs and swing your feet up to the bar and kick off, back to the starting position.

BEGINNERS: 4 sets of 5 reps — with 1 minute break between sets.

INTERMEDIATE: 3 sets of 10 — with 30 seconds break between sets.

1

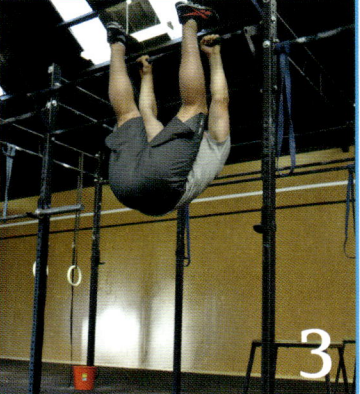
2

3

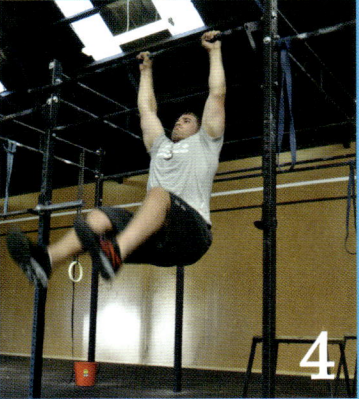
4

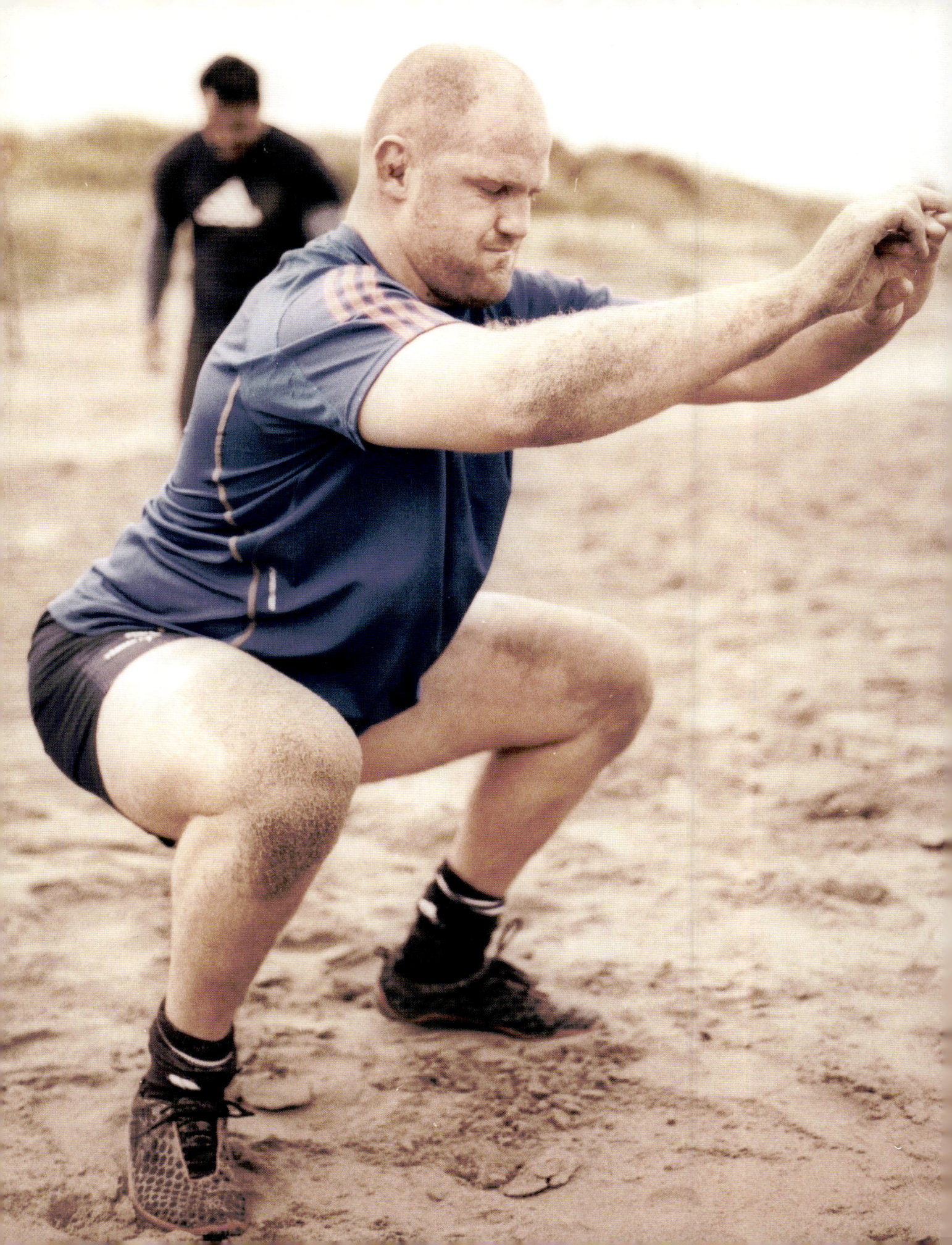

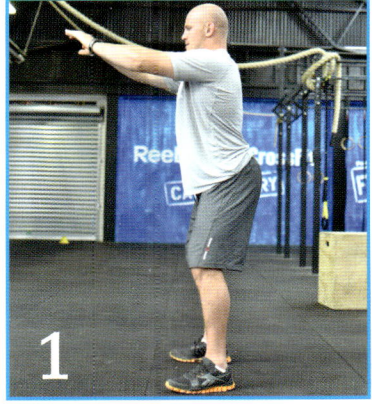

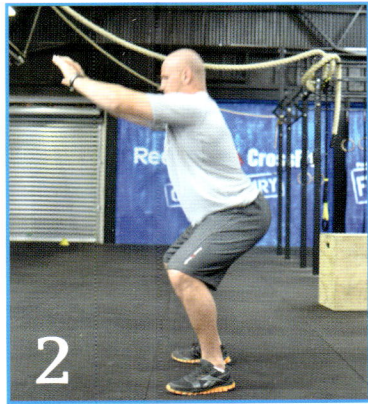

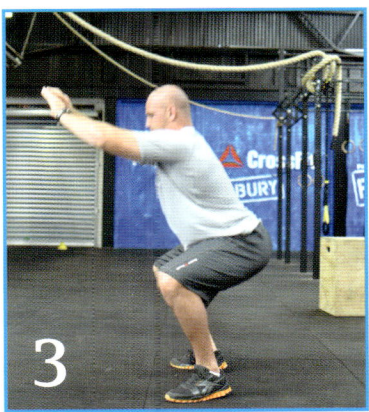

Air squats

Place hands behind your neck or straight out in front, arms extended to ensure an upright body position. Hips dip down at a controlled speed to an imaginary point just below the height of the knees, or as far down before your chest starts to dip forward and lose form. If your chest does dip forward try widening your feet position. And if that doesn't work, go down as far as you can, keeping strict form. With practice your body will adjust and become more flexible. For now all you can do is your best.

BEGINNERS: 20 reps, as fast as you can, before moving on to the next exercise.

INTERMEDIATE: 50 reps, as fast as you can, before moving on to the next exercise.

NOTE: See 'Front squats' on page 95 for a more advanced weighted movement.

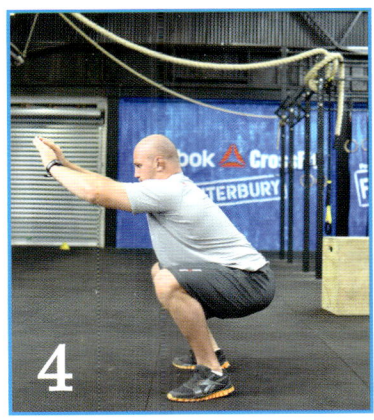

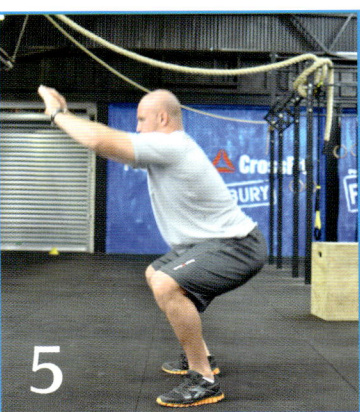

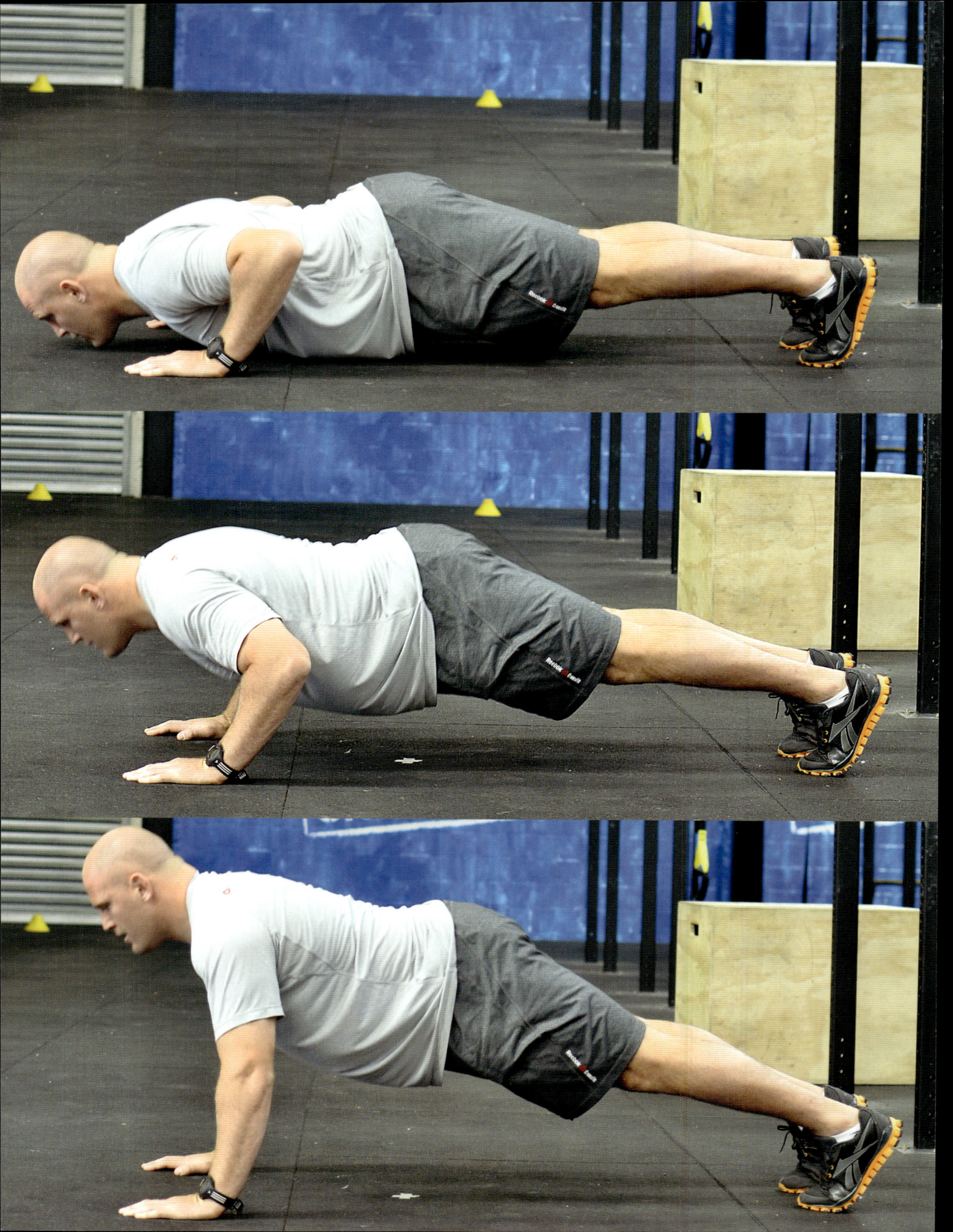

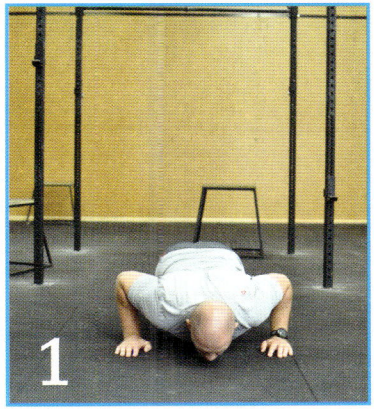

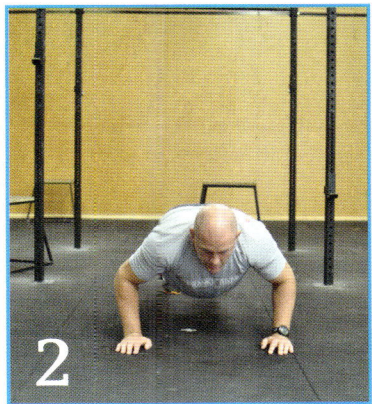

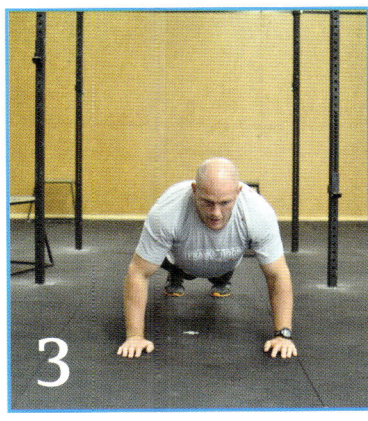

Push-ups

Not only does this basic exercise strengthen the muscles in your chest and arms but it also engages the core and legs. Like a prone hold or bridge (where you support your weight on your elbows and toes), doing strict push-ups strengthens the entire body and is recommended for everybody's training routine. The best thing about them is there is no equipment needed. Try knocking out the Intermediate push-ups right now. It makes for a great warm-up.

BEGINNERS: 10 reps, with your chest touching the ground at the bottom.

INTERMEDIATE: 20 reps, lifting your hands off the ground at the bottom of each rep.

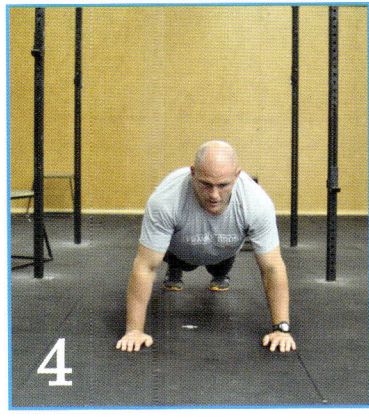

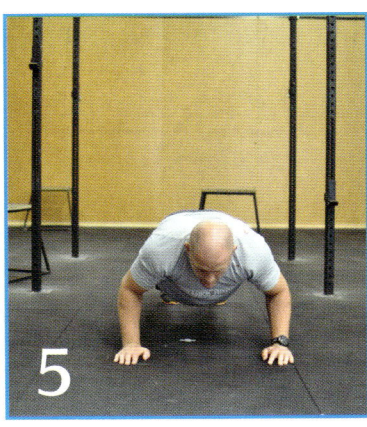

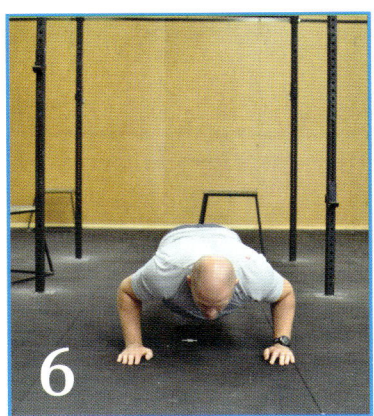

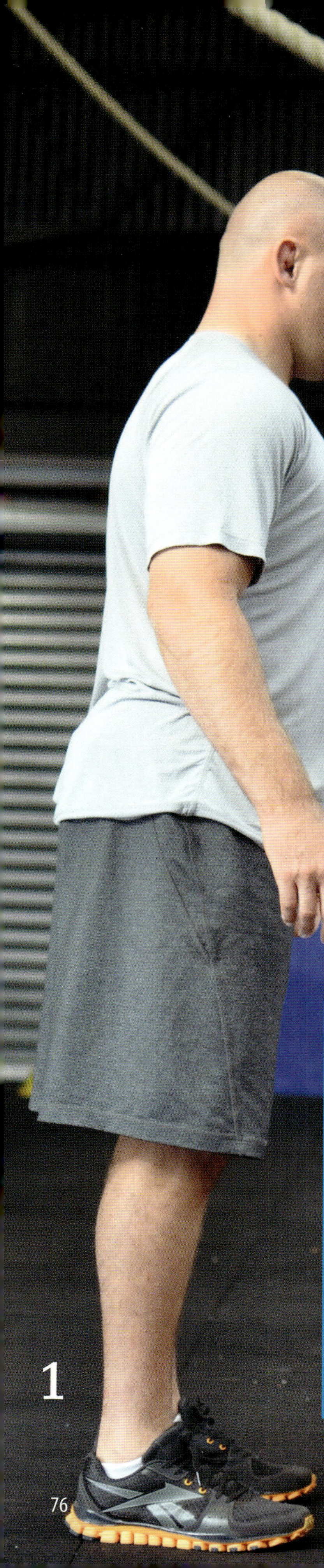

Leg step-ups

A simple exercise designed to strengthen your stride. Concentrate on 100 per cent effort with each lift off the box. Start with one leg on the ground and the other leg bent on the box, bench or chair. Focus on the quads, located above your knee. With one leg, step up onto the box. Stand up straight, with both legs on top of the box, then hop down. Alternate legs.

BEGINNER: 12 each leg.

INTERMEDIATE: 25 each leg.

1

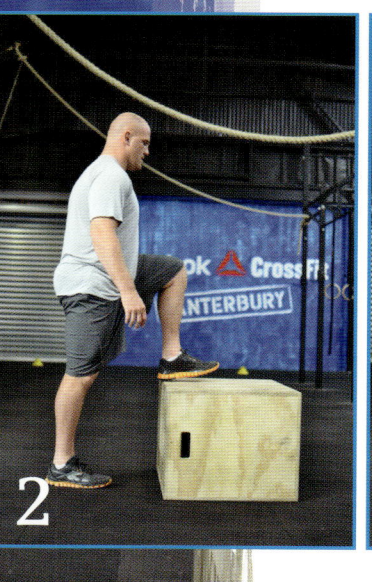

2

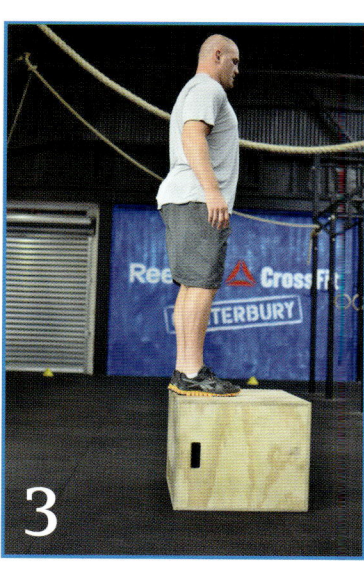

3

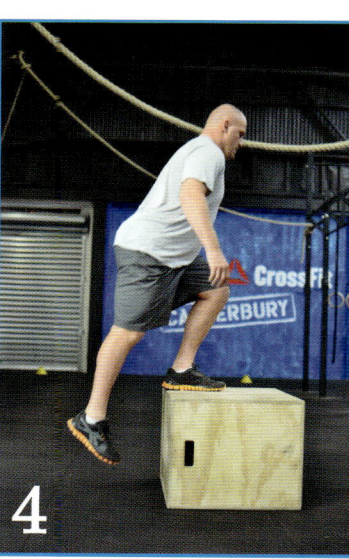

4

Chin-ups & Pull-ups

A chin-up has a narrow grip with your palms facing towards you and is a good exercise for beginners who need to build some early strength in their back muscles. A pull-up has a wider grip with the palm of the hand facing away from you. This is harder than the chin-up and is one of the best exercises for developing the muscles of the back.

BEGINNERS: 6 reps, using an underhand or overhand grip.

INTERMEDIATE: 12 reps, using a wider underhand or overhand grip.

Chin-ups

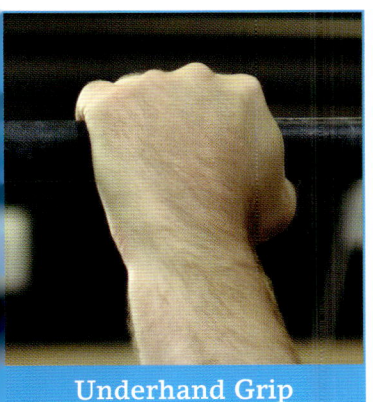

Underhand Grip

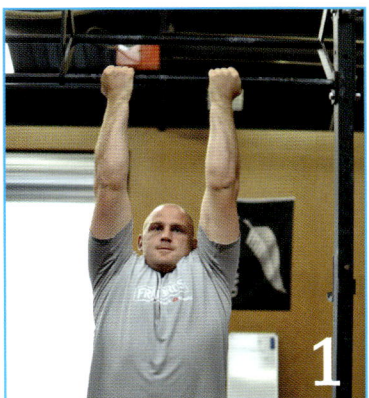

1

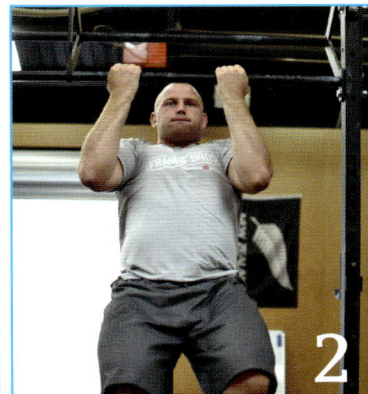

2

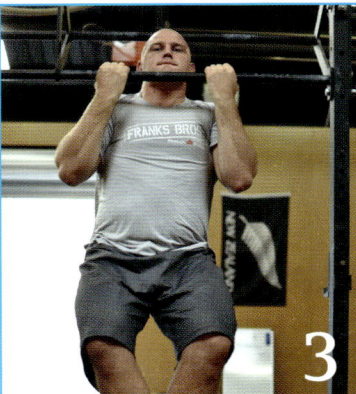

3

Pull-ups

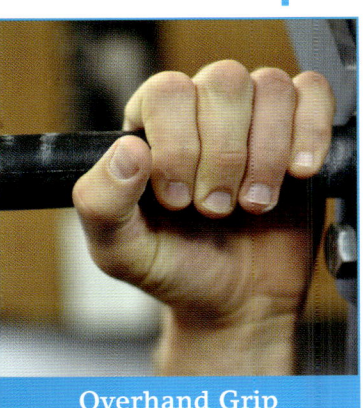

Overhand Grip

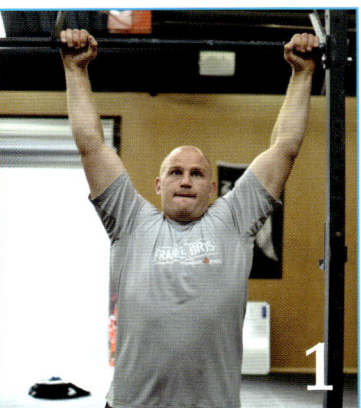

1

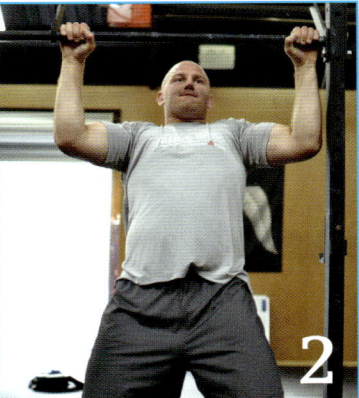

2

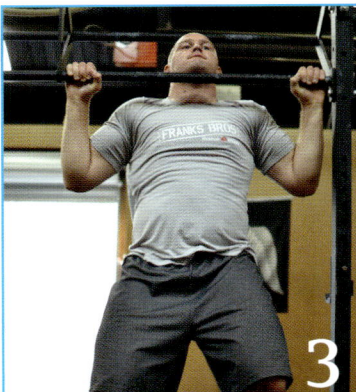

3

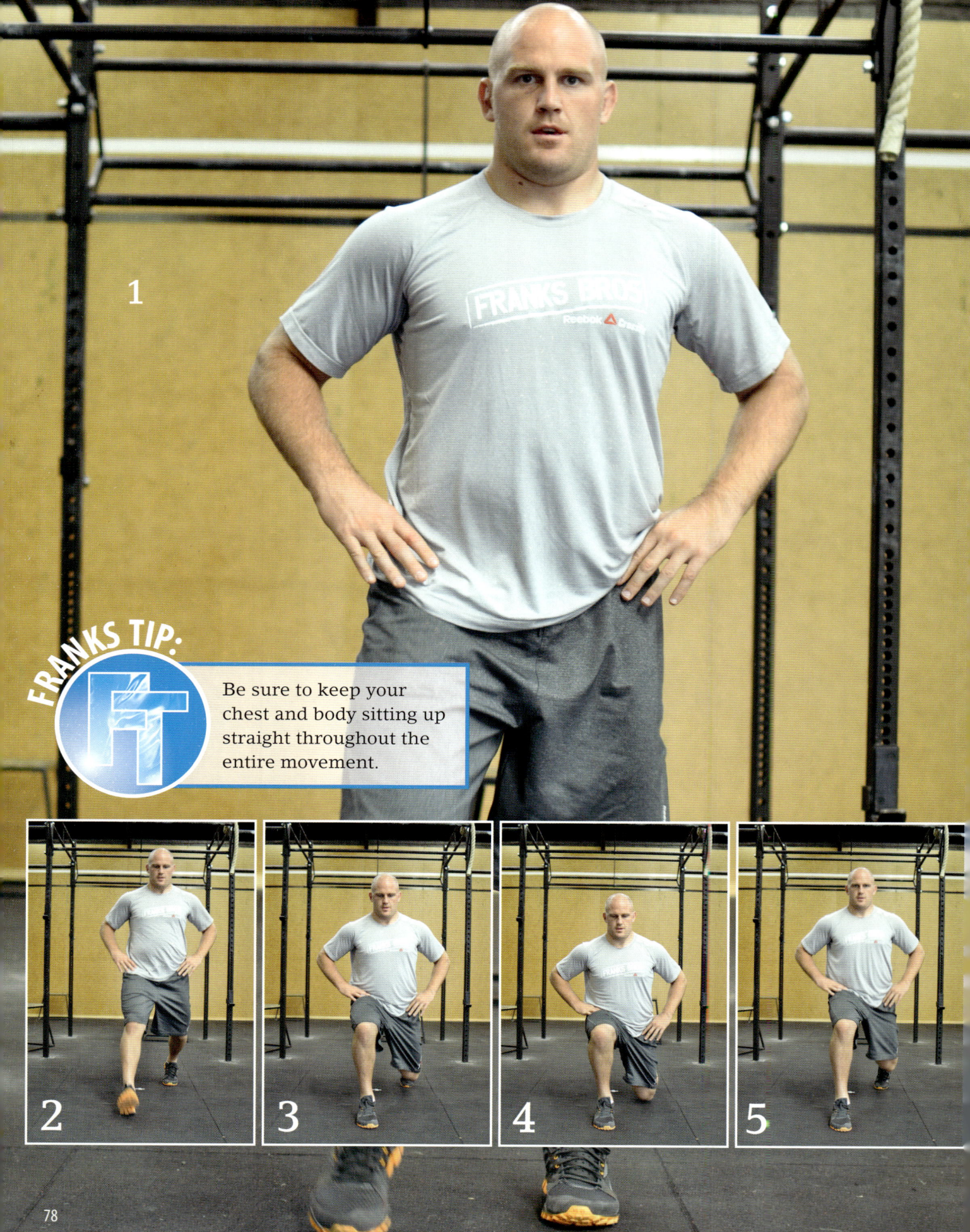

1

2

3

4

5

Lunges

Fundamental to any leg workout, lunges can be done on the spot or around the room and with or without weighted dumbbells. At the end of each set ideally the muscles located at the top of your legs should have a slight sensation of burning. The Franks brothers like to get to that sensation of burning by halfway through the exercise and learn to keep pushing through the 'good pain' to really stress their muscles to grow.

Start (and finish) standing straight up with your feet together. Step forward so your front leg bends 90 degrees, allowing your back knee to lightly touch the ground. Then using all the speed and power possible either return to the starting position or step through, focusing on the muscles in the bent leg.

BEGINNER: 10 lunges on each leg.

INTERMEDIATE: 10 lunges on each leg, while holding a 10 kg plate.

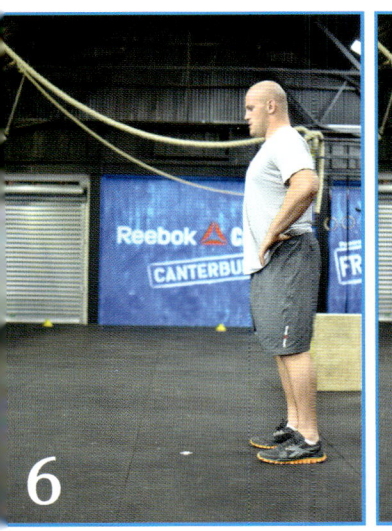
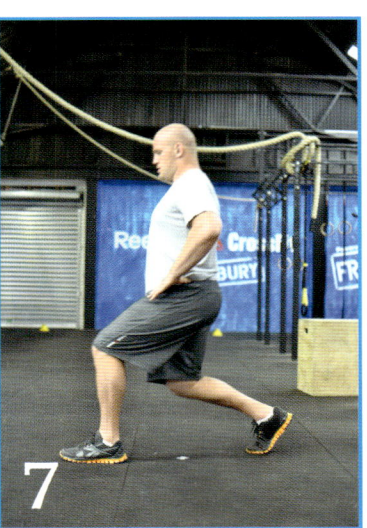
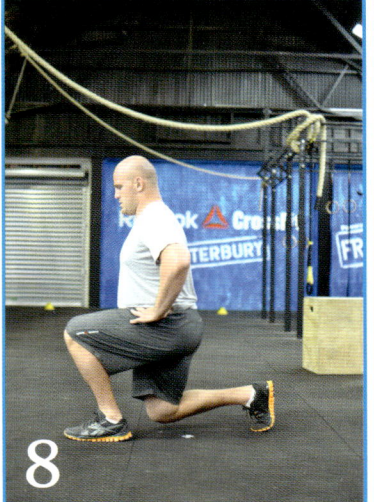
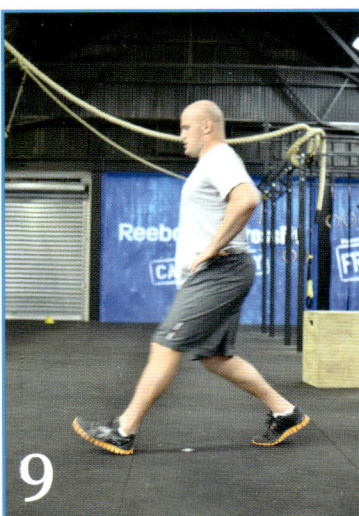

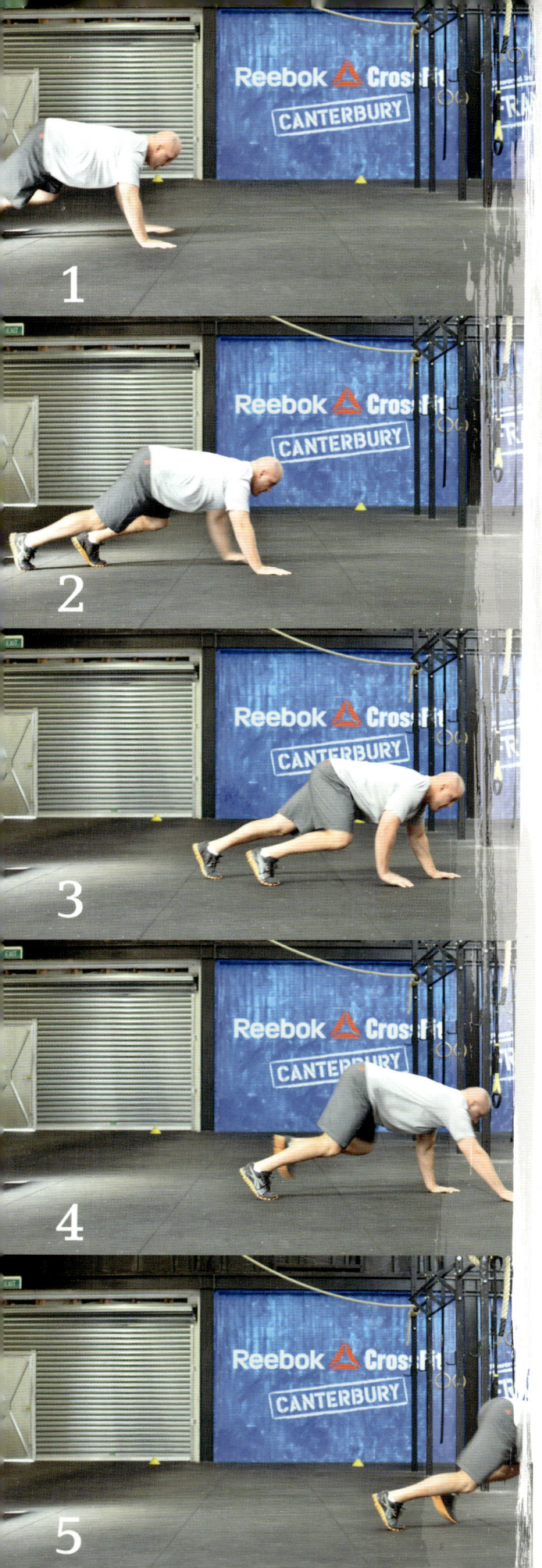

Bear crawl

A typical military or pre-season team drill, the bear crawl is a full-body workout that can quickly warm up the arms and shoulders.

Bending 90 degrees at the hips, place your hands on the ground and run while distributing your body weight evenly between your arms and legs.

BEGINNERS: Crawl in any direction, non-stop, for 60 seconds, keeping on your hands and knees.

INTERMEDIATE:
A) Crawl 10 metres forward and 10 metres backwards.
B) Crawl 10 metres right and 10 metres left.

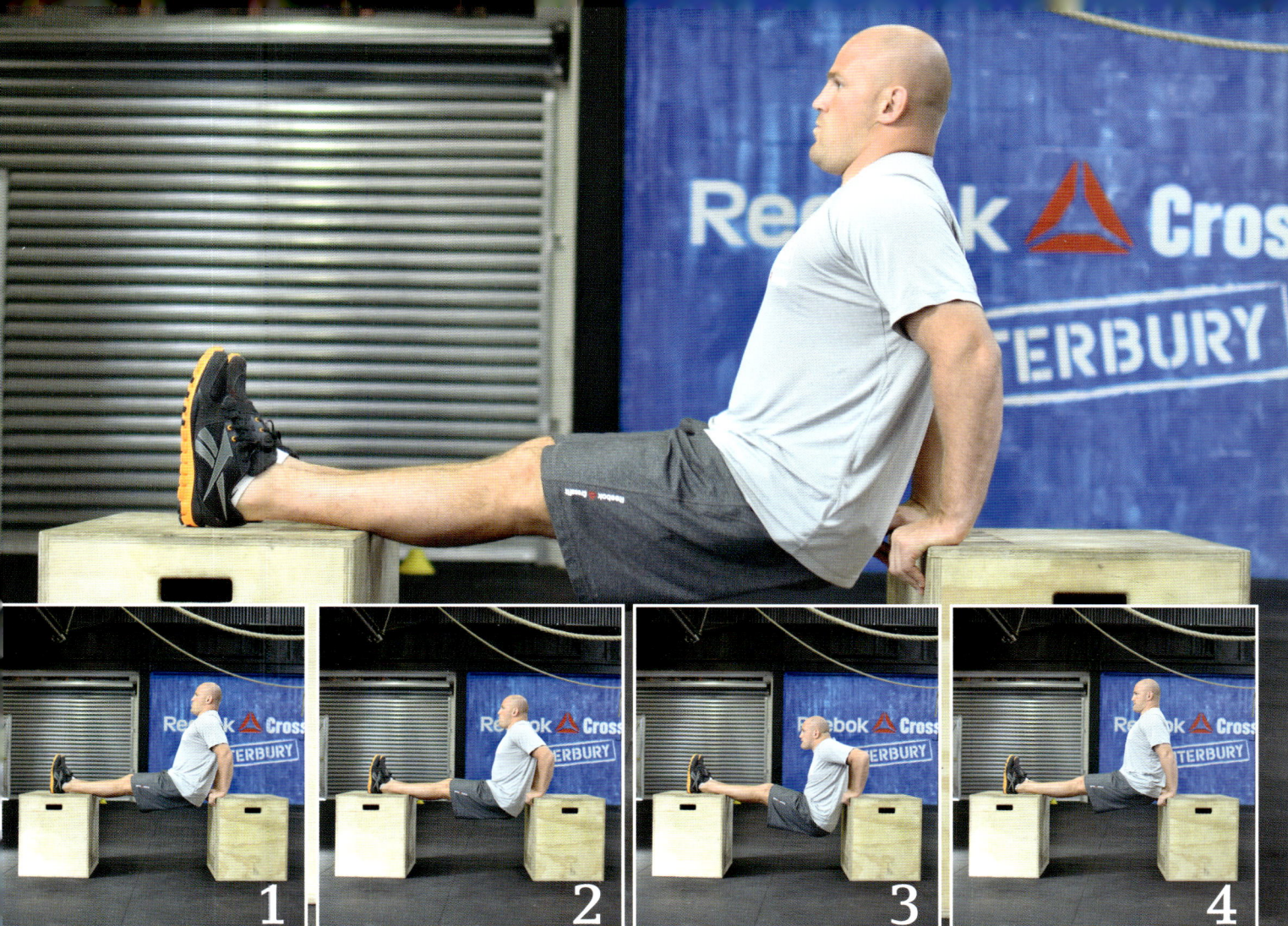

Triceps dip

The largest arm muscle group is the triceps and this muscle usually responds well to direct loading.

Using a bench, box, or step, place your hands behind your hips and extend your legs forward. Transfer as much body weight to your arms, then lower your body by bending your arms 90 degrees. Keep your body rigid. Extend your arms back out to the starting position, then repeat.

BEGINNER: 10 reps, with your feet on the floor and your hands behind you on a box (or bench), before moving on to the next exercise.

INTERMEDIATE: 15 reps, with your feet elevated on top of a box or bench (see photo) to put more resistance on your arms, before moving on to the next exercise.

Lateral slides

This is a very important exercise to help with your lateral movement — in other words your ability to move quickly left or right. With bent knees, hands out in front of you to help with balance and chest upright, move as quickly as you can sideways and try not to let your feet cross. Lateral slides will strengthen the muscles required to change direction and contribute to an athlete's agility.

For beginners, a flat space 10 metres wide will do. For intermediate athletes, finding a steep hill to slip up and down on will add much more resistance for the slide. Gravity will apply more of your own body weight back onto your leg muscles. Then after a day or two of recovery this exercise will have helped you become a lot more explosive.

BEGINNER: Slide 10 metres left side, then 10 metres right side.

INTERMEDIATE: Slide 10 metres up and down a steep hill, then turn and face the opposite direction and repeat.

Hill sprints

Running up a hill is not rocket science, but there is some positive physics to illustrate.

The steeper the hill, the more resistance gravity will apply to your body – not to mention the more explosive your body will become.

BEGINNER: Sprint 20 metres up a steep hill as fast as you can and then walk back down.

INTERMEDIATE: Sprint 60 metres up a steep hill and jog back down.

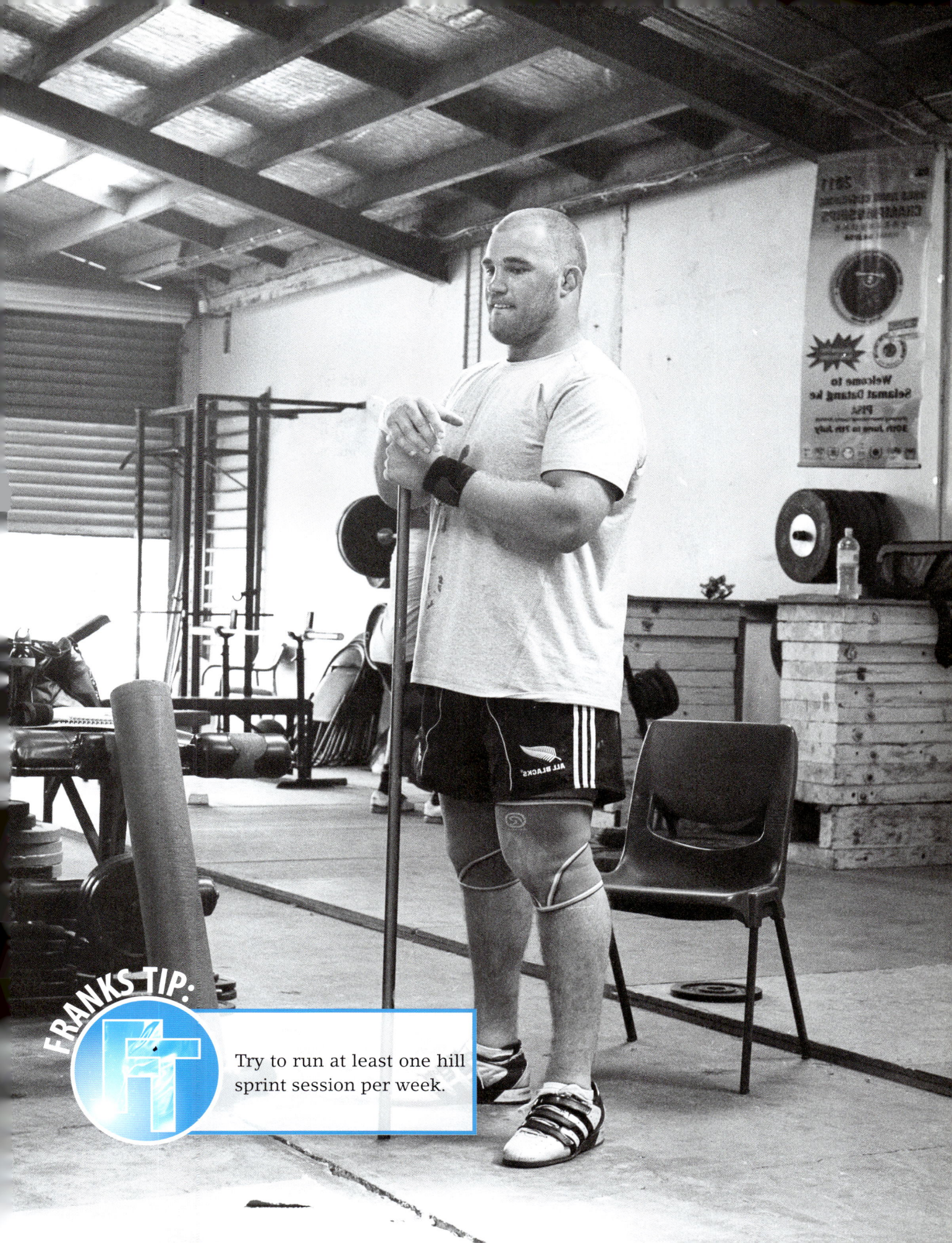

FRANKS TIP:

Try to run at least one hill sprint session per week.

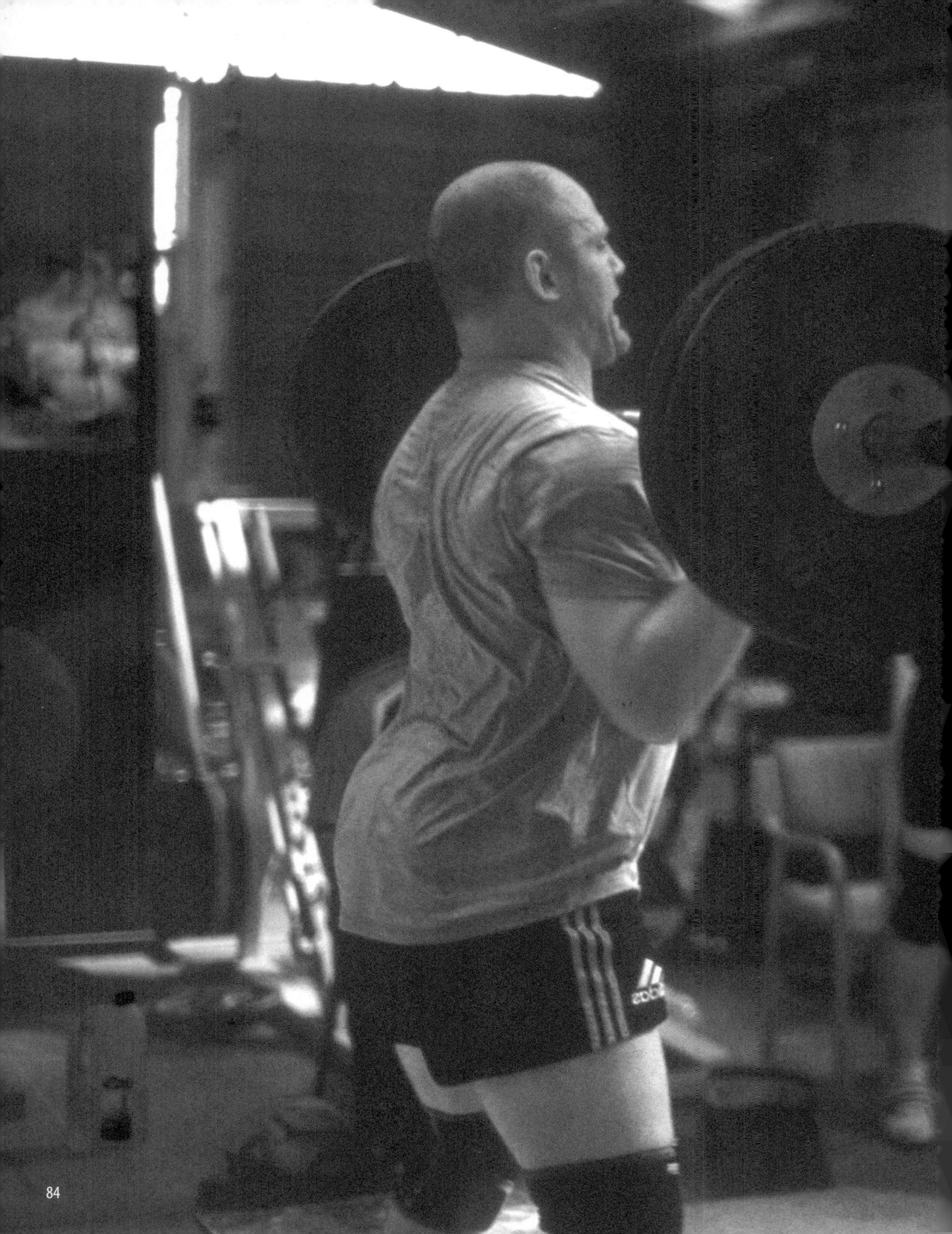

WEIGHTED EXERCISES

Before doing any weight training, make sure you are fully warmed up and loose. When training with weights a decision needs to be made about what kind of muscle the athlete wants to grow. Training with heavier weights that only allow the muscles to repeat any given movement once or twice will produce a different result than training with a lighter weight that can be repeated 10 to 15 times quickly. If you are new to weight training a good target weight should allow you to do 10 repetitions.

The exercises featured in this book are but a few ways to target the various muscle groups in the body. As an athlete moves from gym to gym other techniques can be learned just by observing others in training or by asking for on-the-spot advice. The internet is also a great tool for learning more methods. Whatever you try you should stick with what gets the best results or at least the most satisfaction. Learning new ways to challenge the body helps you stay motivated and offers a better overall result. Simply use the following exercises as a base before specialising.

If you don't have all the right equipment for one or more of the featured workouts, don't fret. Simply replace it with a similar exercise or find the equivalent bodyweight exercise and increase the reps. For example, if you don't have a lateral pulldown machine, try doing 3 sets of 10 overhand pull-ups.

There are always hundreds of excuses why not to exercise. The hardest part is getting your shoes tied up and making it out the front door.

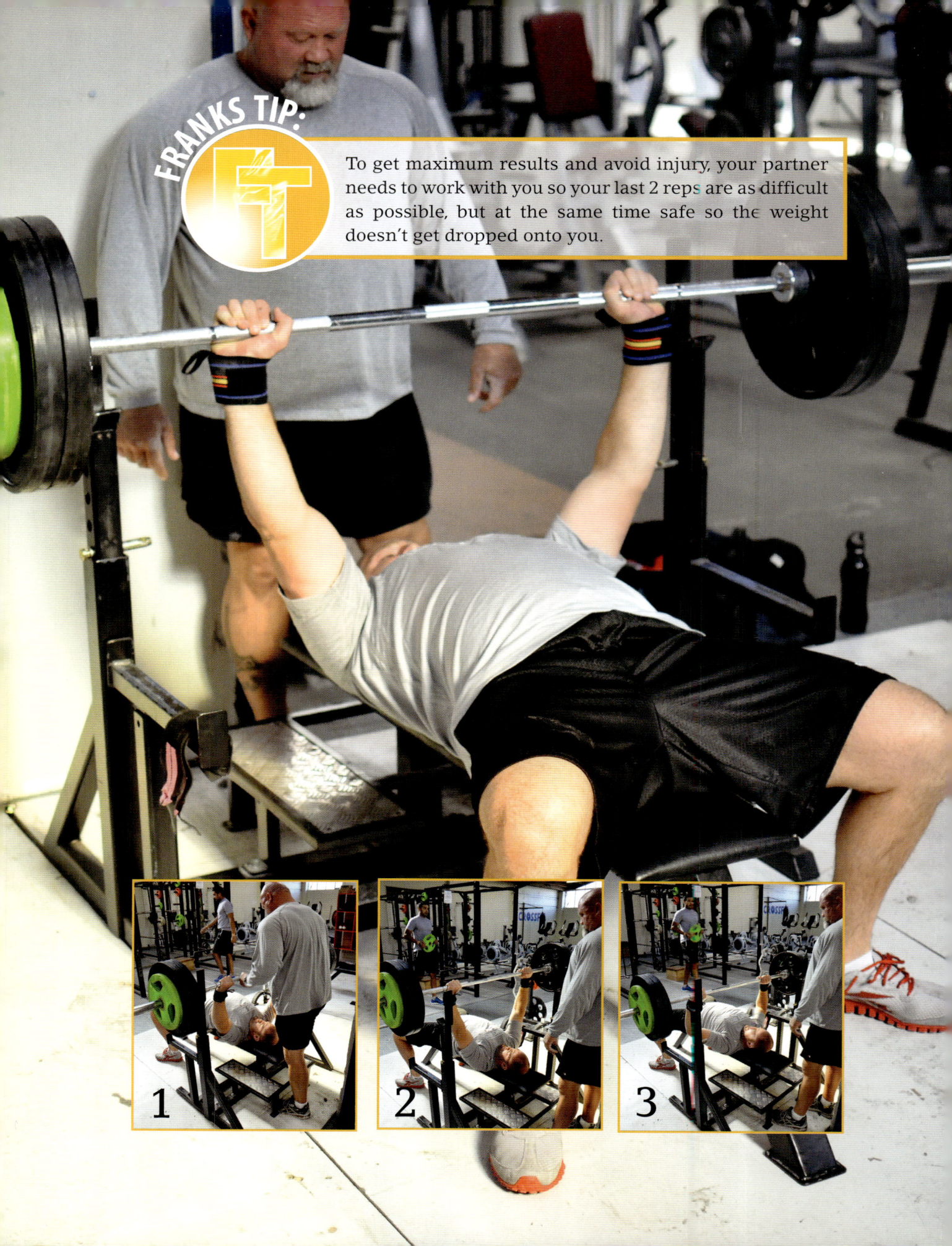

FRANKS TIP:

To get maximum results and avoid injury, your partner needs to work with you so your last 2 reps are as difficult as possible, but at the same time safe so the weight doesn't get dropped onto you.

1

2

3

Bench press

The bench press is a common powerlifting exercise used to target the arms and chest. For some unknown reason, it is common for athletes to measure their opponents' strength based on what weight they can bench press. Maybe it is due to the fact that bench press is one of the few exercises where a partner is mandatory. Especially when lifting a heavy weight, ask someone nearby to 'spot you'.

If you don't have a bench, use the floor. If you don't have a bar, use a pair of dumbbells. The position of your hands changes which of the two main muscle groups are mainly being used. A very wide grip targets the chest, while a narrow grip increases the height of the bar and targets the arms. Get your partner to help get the weight into position. Lower the bar, remembering the path is NOT straight down, but a smooth arc down towards your body's centre, then back up over the chest.

To build a balanced body, when training any muscle group, it is very important to add an additional exercise to work the opposite muscles. This is called a 'super set'. In this case, match the intensity of your bench press workout with a back exercise such as the dumbbell row (see page 99).

BEGINNER: 3 sets of 10 reps. Start the first set so you can do 10 reps easily. Finish the last set of 10 with a weight which makes it difficult to finish the final rep.

INTERMEDIATE: 3 sets of 8 reps. Start the first set so you can do 8 reps on your own. Finish the last set of 8 with a weight that requires help from your partner on the final rep.

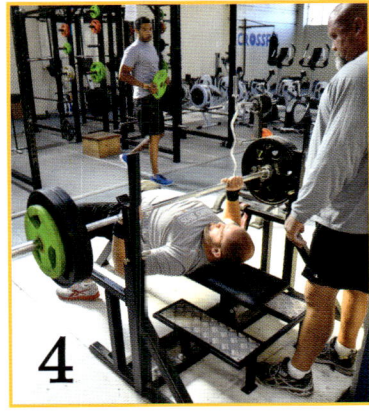
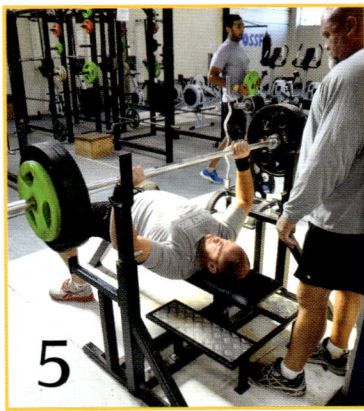
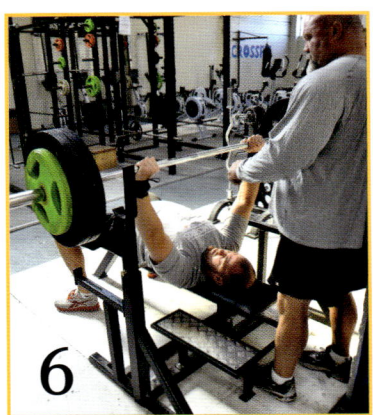

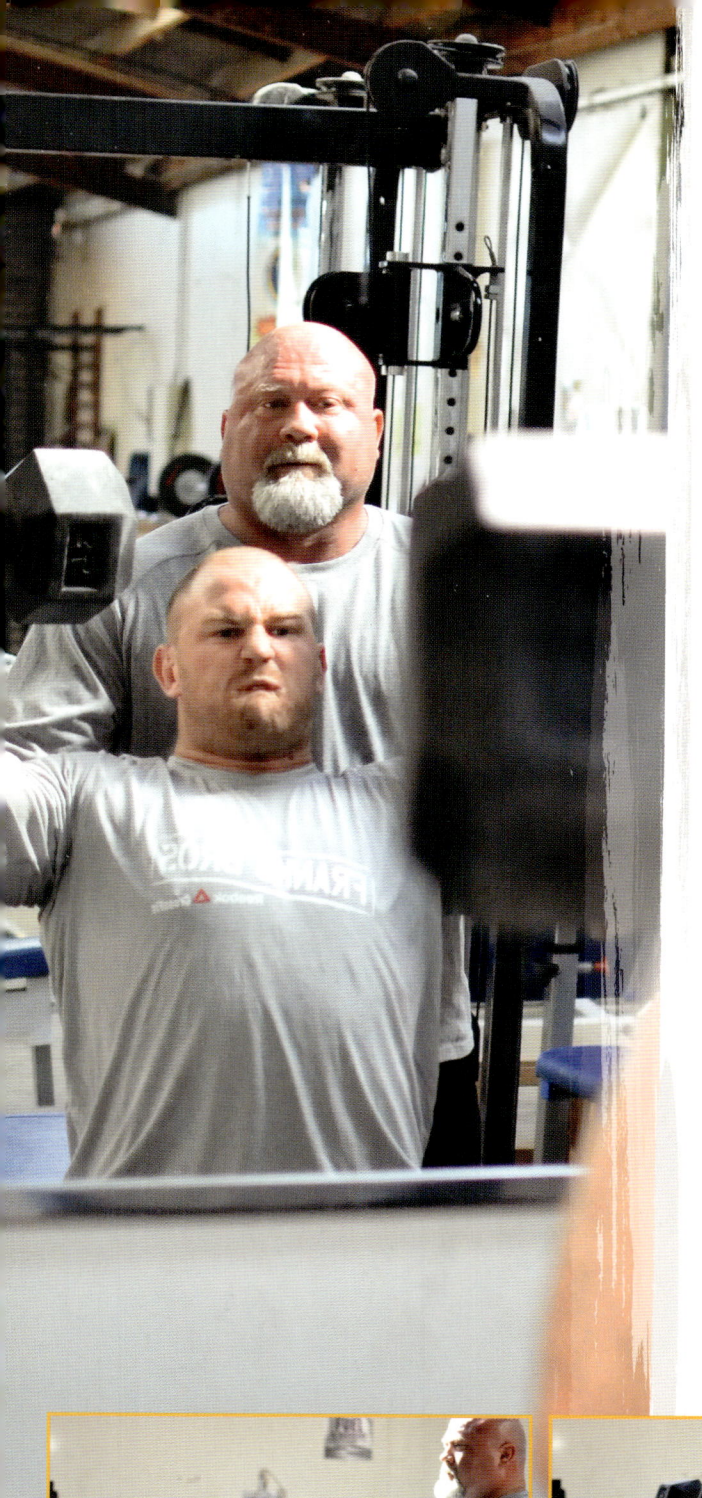

Seated shoulder press

This basic shoulder exercise is a great way to build and strengthen the various muscles that make up your shoulders. As your body develops through training, other shoulder exercises can be added. When starting out, however, the seated shoulder press exercise is fundamental. If you don't have any suitable dumbbells you can use a barbell instead. Even if you use the bar with no added plates, begin with a weight that you can only just achieve 12 to 15 reps, then add 1 to 2 kg each week as your shoulders strengthen.

Start with the hands turned out, elbows out to your side, bent to 90 degrees. Press dumbbells upwards, straightening the elbows and finishing with your arms straight above your head.

BEGINNER: Find a weight that you can lift no more than 15 reps, 3 sets.

INTERMEDIATE: Lift a heavier weight that you can only repeat 10 reps, 4 sets.

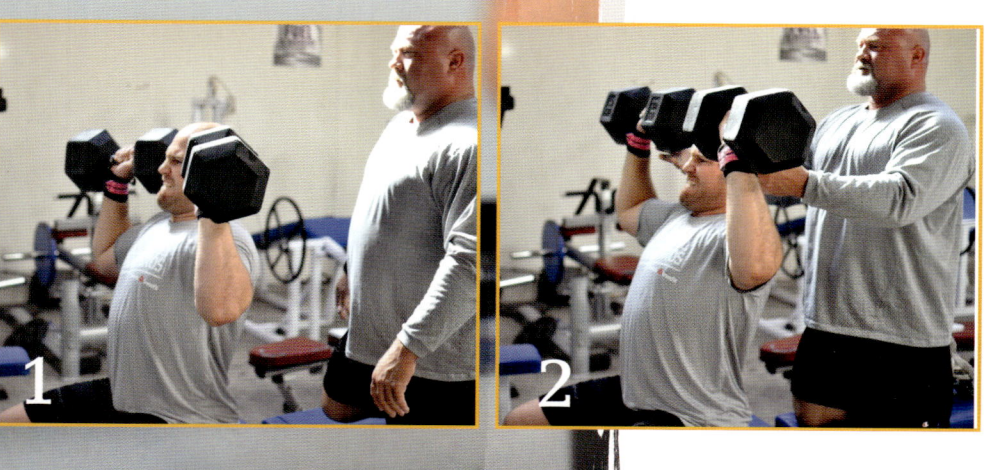

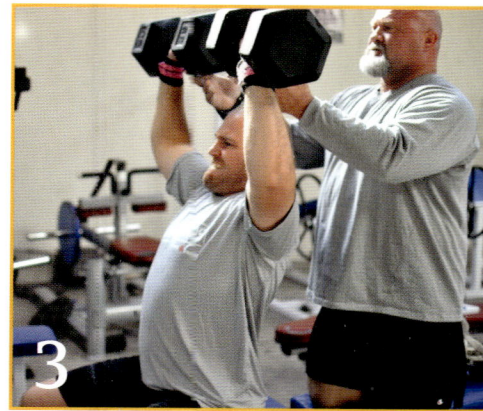

Lateral pull-downs

Regardless of what shaped handle features on the end of the pulley, the lat pulldown is an excellent exercise for isolating the wing-shaped muscles on the side of your body as well as working the majority of the powerful back muscles. The muscles used in this exercise help pull your body closer to your arms as when climbing a rope, and will also give you more overall arm strength and control.

For the first set start by pinning the weight into the machine (if you don't know the weight, start with half of your own body weight) and set up the machine seat height and leg-lock position. Sit up in a straight angle (as demonstrated by Ben below). Hold that same body angle as you pull the weight down as low as your elbows will allow. Control the weight back up to just before the arms are in a fully locked position. Then repeat.

BEGINNER: Keeping your back in the same position, find a weight that you can lift 10 reps for 3 sets.

INTERMEDIATE: Increasing weight on each set, lift a heavier weight so you are struggling to finish 8 reps, 3 sets.

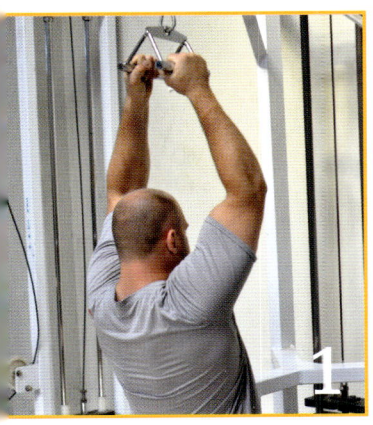 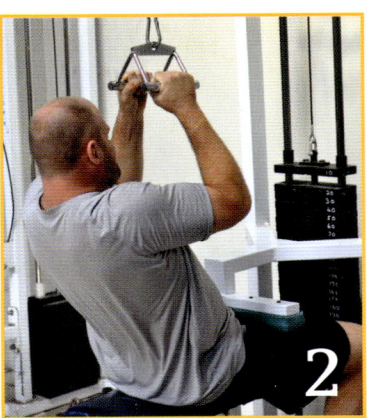 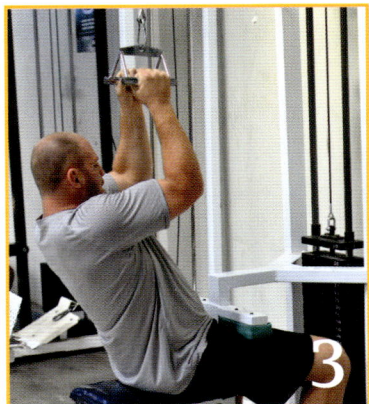 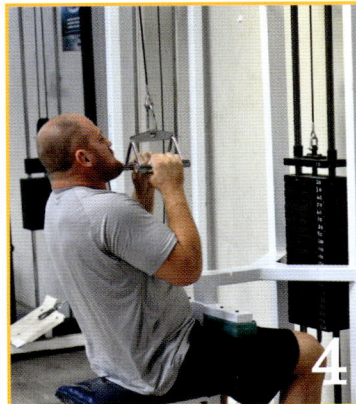

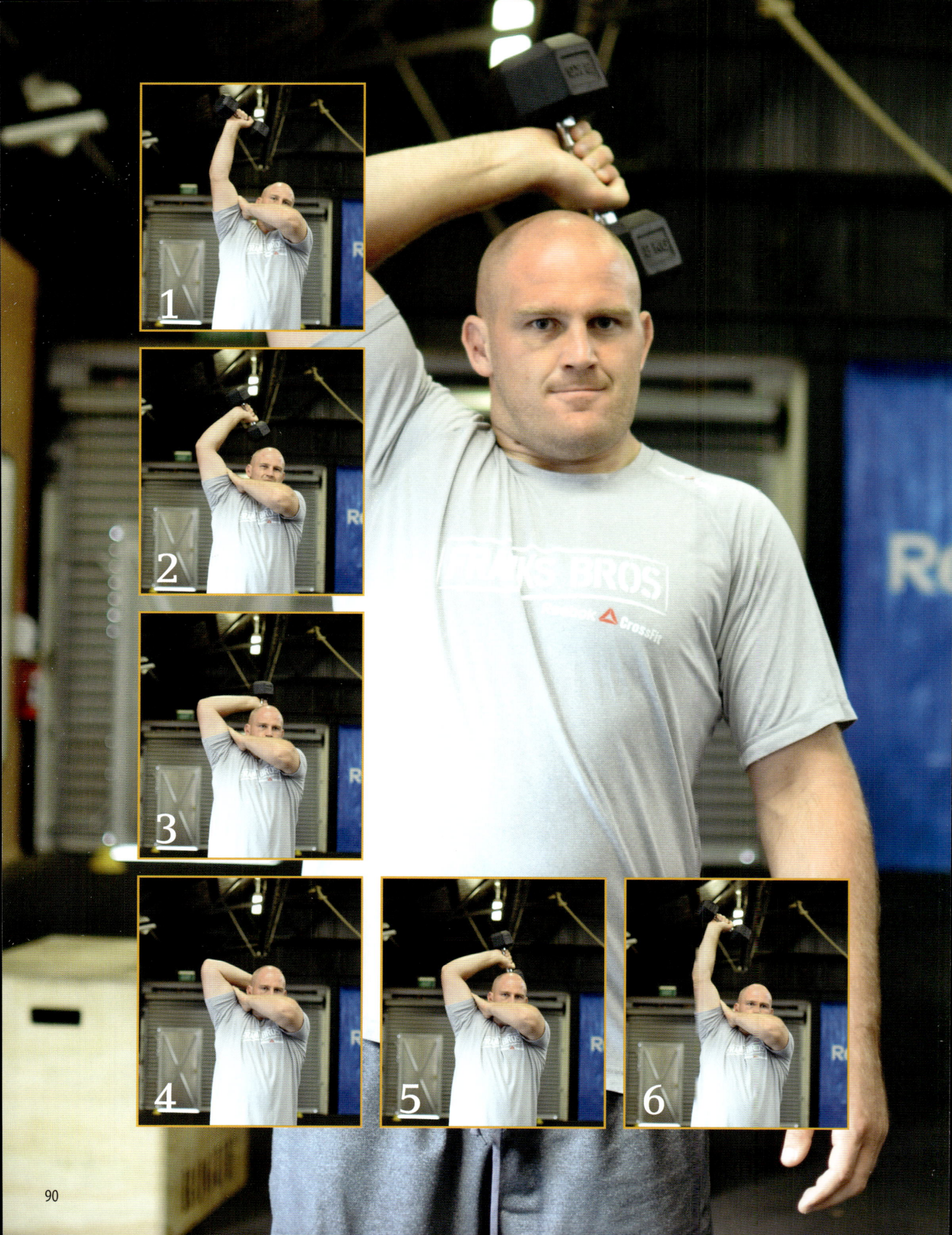

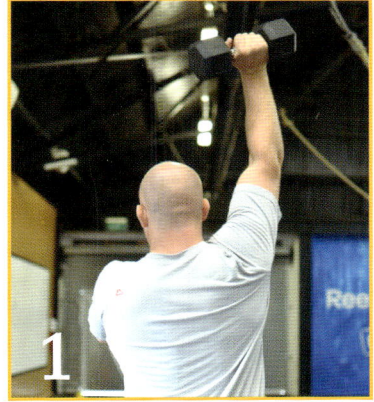

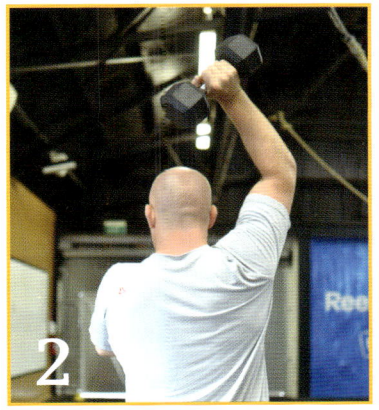

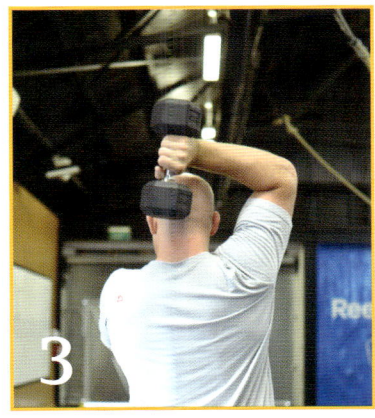

Triceps extensions

Great for building up strength in the arms, this exercise targets the largest arm muscle group, the triceps.

Working one arm at a time, find a suitable dumbbell weight – 5 or 10 kg is a good start. Hold the weight behind your head, supporting your shoulders with your opposite hand. Hammer the weight upwards in an arc shape and slowly return the weight back down through the same path to the start position and repeat.

BEGINNER: Find a weight that you can lift no more than 15 reps, 3 sets.

INTERMEDIATE: Lift a heavier weight that you can only just manage to repeat 10 reps, 4 sets.

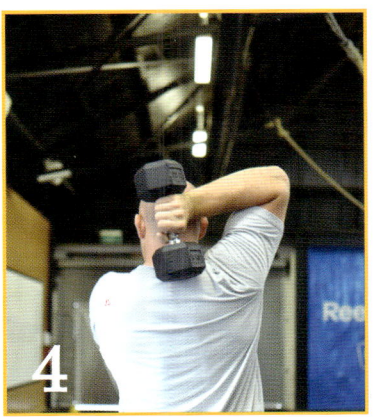

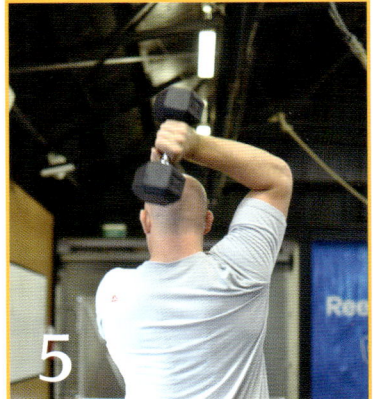

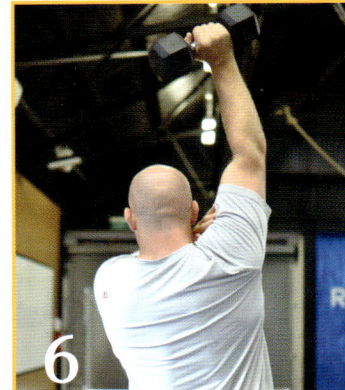

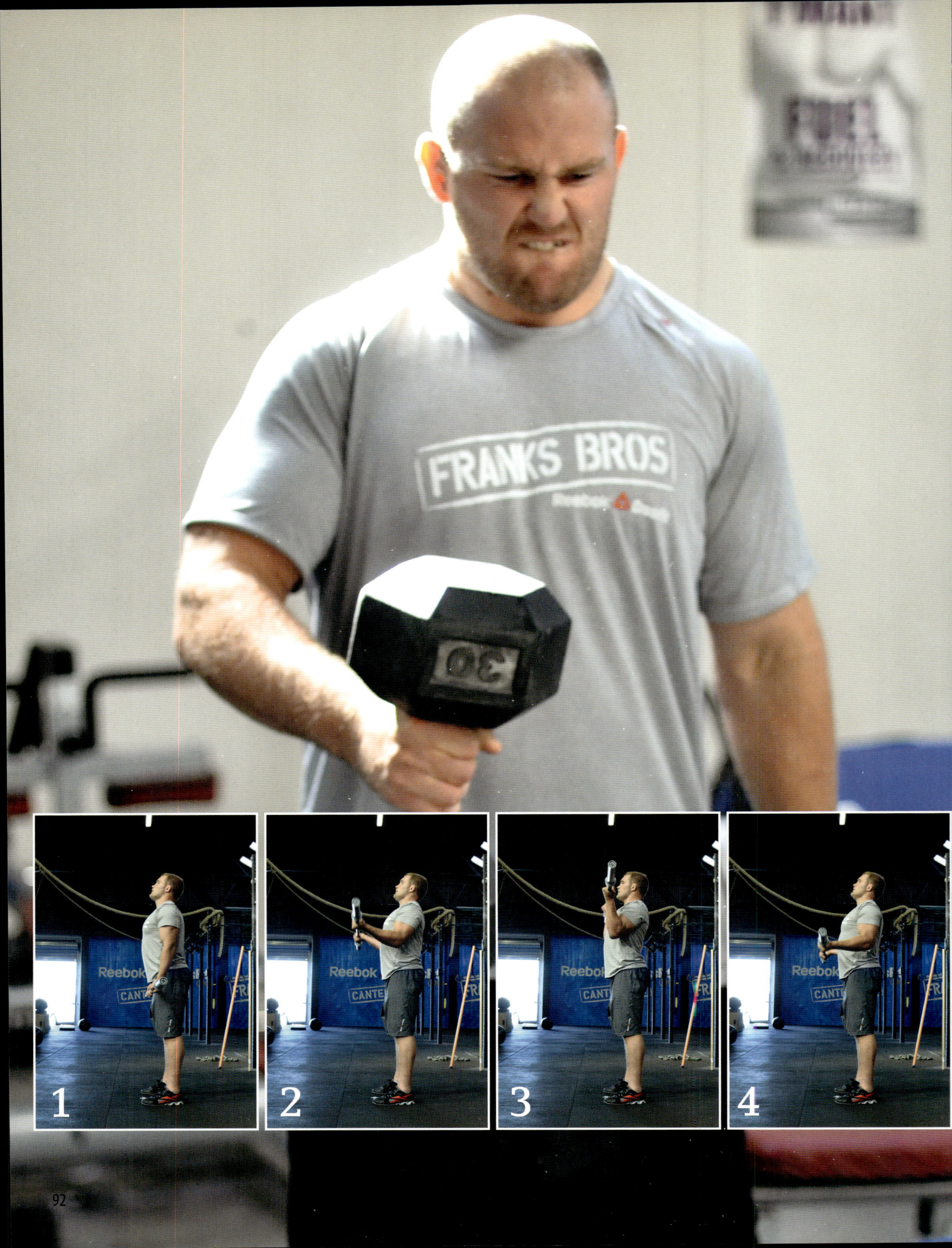

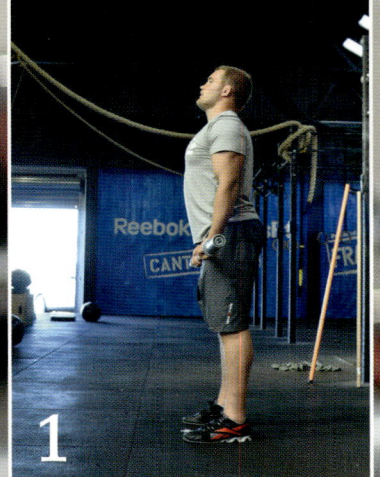
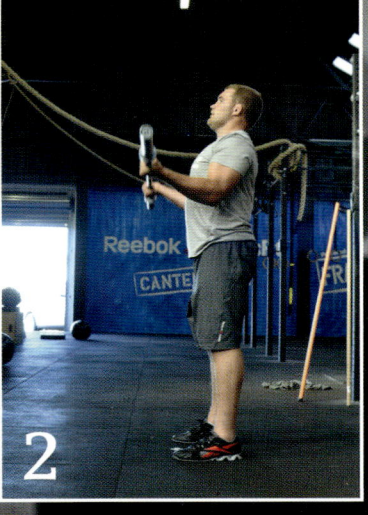
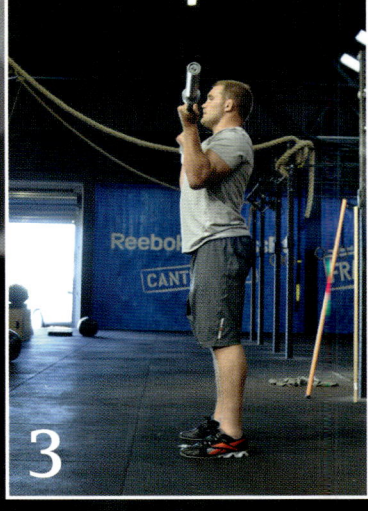
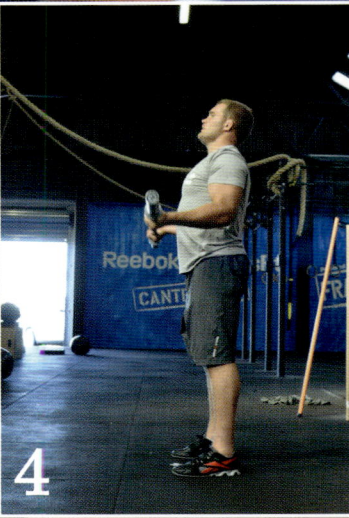

Biceps curls

Used to strengthen the curling motion of your arms, curls can be done with either a weighted bar or a set of dumbbells. It is important to find a weight that you can lift with your bicep muscles alone, and not swing your body or hips to help each curl. If nothing else, a set of large biceps will intimidate your opponent before the whistle even starts!

Stand up tall with your feet comfortably set and hands shoulder-width apart. Bending from the elbows, curl the weight up and down, alternating if you have dumbbells.

BEGINNER: Find a weight that you can lift no more than 15 reps, 3 sets.

INTERMEDIATE: Lift a heavier weight that you can only repeat 10 reps, 4 sets.

FRANKS TIP:

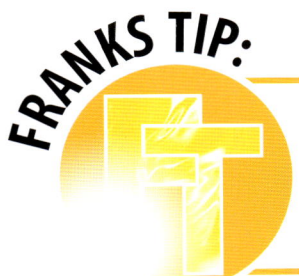

Stand up tall and focus on strictly working the arms without swinging your body about.

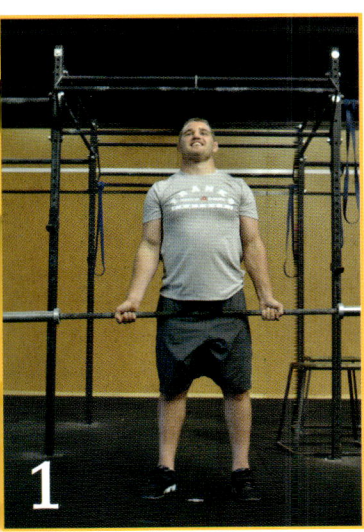
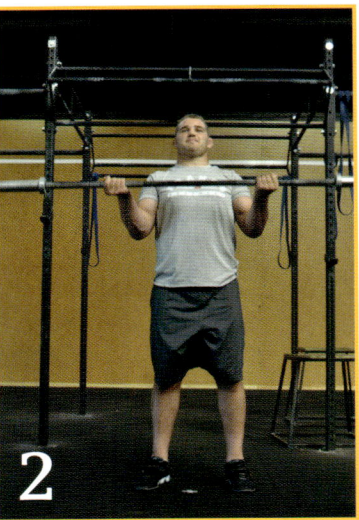
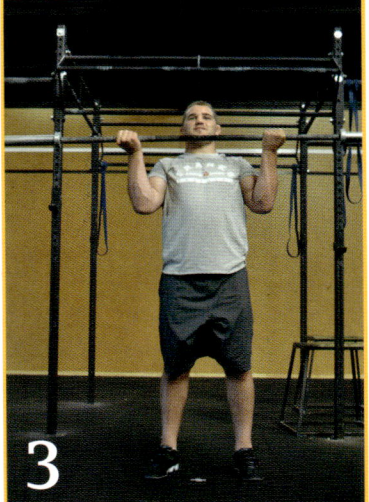
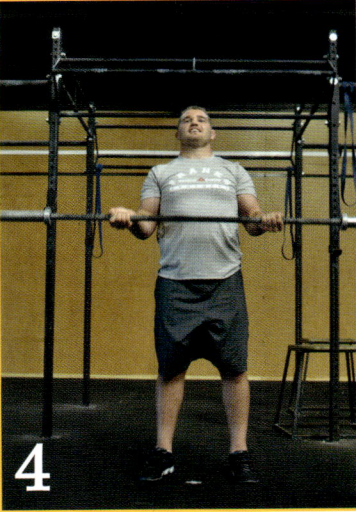

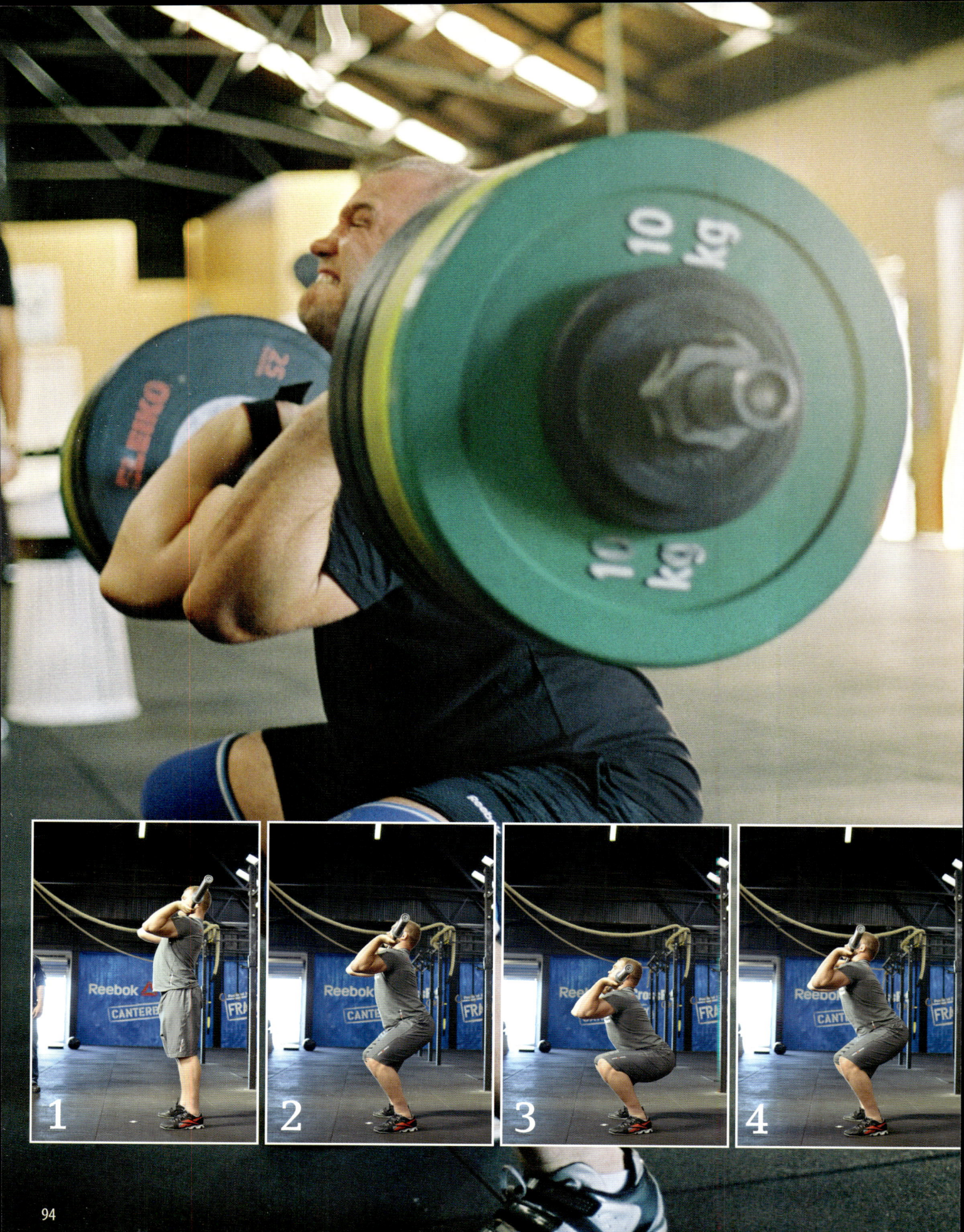

Front squat

Athletes with less flexibility in their hips and ankles prefer the front squat to the big brother back squat. When attempting a front squat less load is placed on the back and hamstring muscle groups; more focus, however, is placed on the front of the legs. Foot position can range between wide to shoulder-width apart. If new to the exercise, start and warm up with the bar with no weights. 'Rack' the bar across the front of the shoulders, with your elbows up high. Weight on the heels, lower at the knees, keeping your chest up. Go down low, or until you feel your chest starting to dip forward. Ideally, go down to a deep squat. Stay strong at the bottom of the movement and don't relax or bounce. Focusing on keeping your elbows up high, drive the bar back up to a standing position.

BEGINNER: Find a weight that you can lift no more than 15 reps, 3 sets.

INTERMEDIATE: Lift a heavier weight that you can only repeat 10 reps, 4 sets.

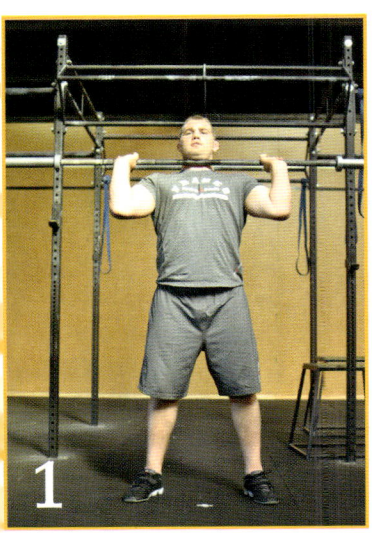
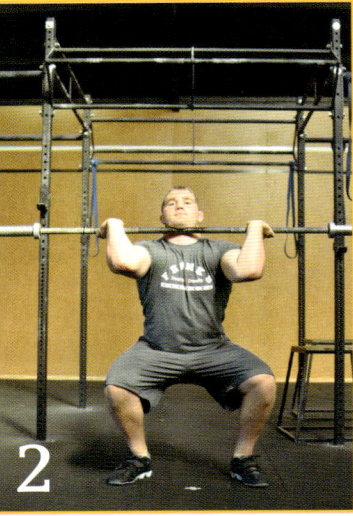
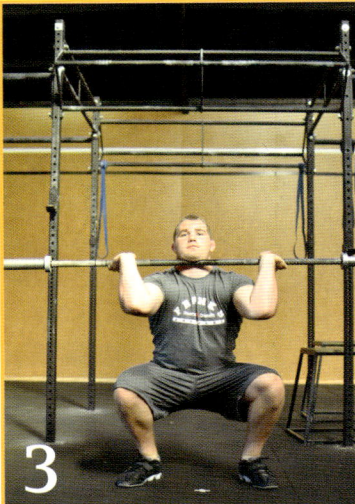
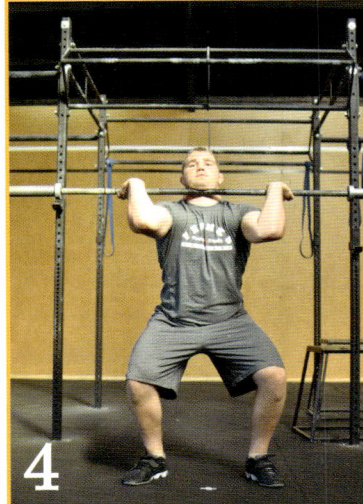

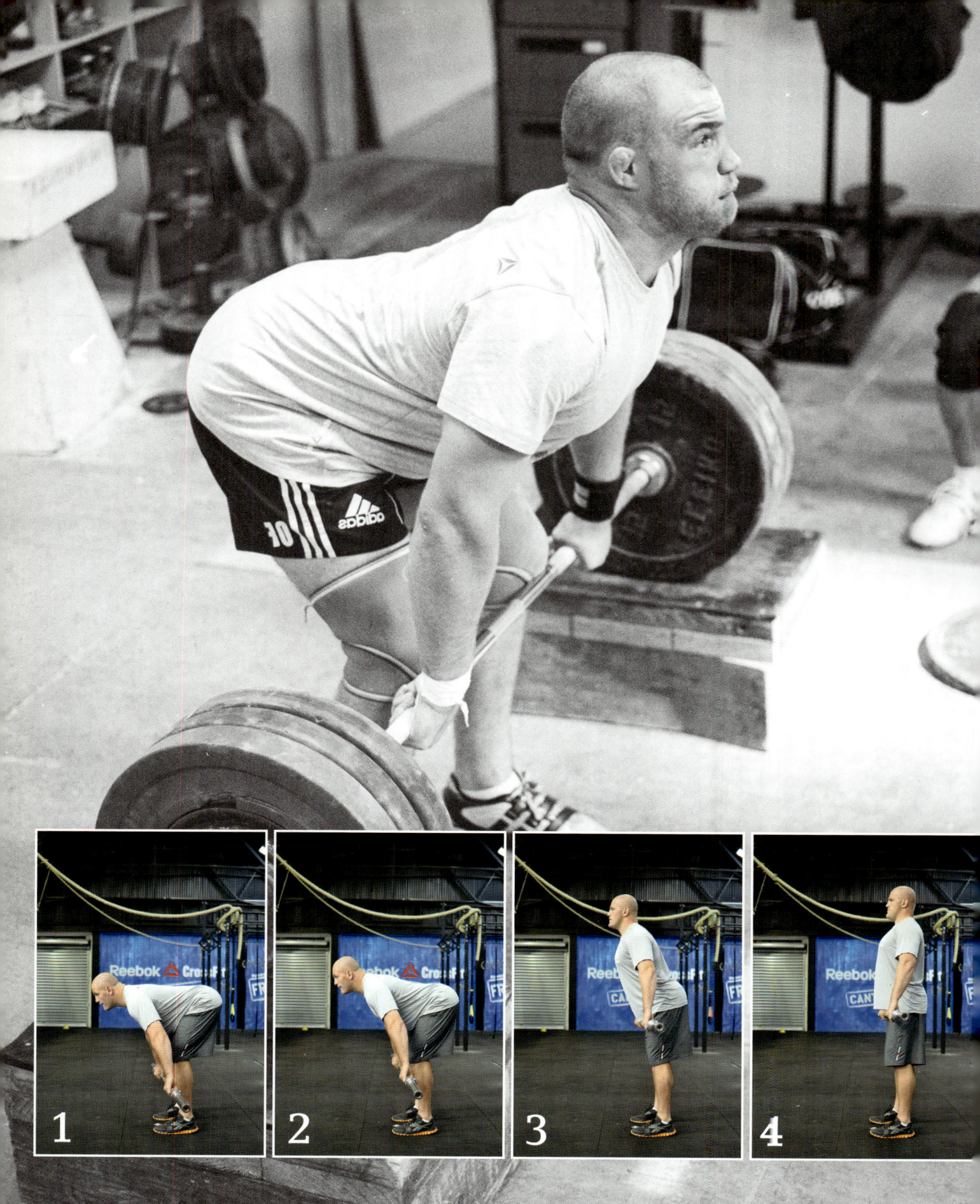

Romanian dead lift

Because the dead lift requires the combined strength of every muscle in the back of your body, it is very important to get the posture and technique right. With your feet shoulder-width apart, bend at the knees and hips and grab the bar. Overhand grip slightly wider than your hips. Before you engage the lift, make sure you are on the heels of your feet and that you can wiggle your toes. Drive the bar up from the floor, keeping your back arched while emphasising your bum and hips. Finish by standing up straight with your shoulders back.

BEGINNER: Find a weight that you can lift no more than 15 reps, 3 sets.

INTERMEDIATE: Lift a heavier weight that you can only repeat 10 reps, 4 sets.

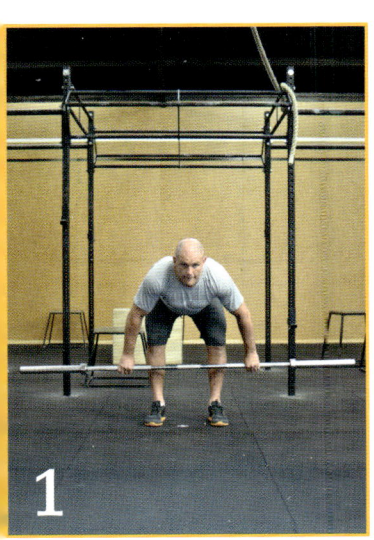
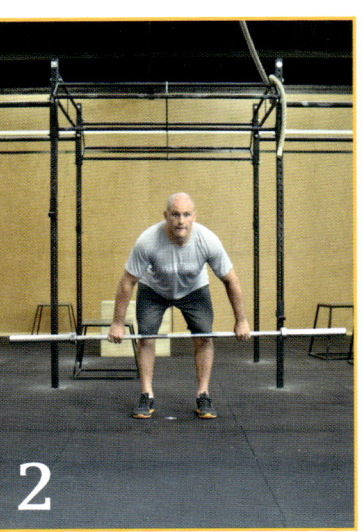
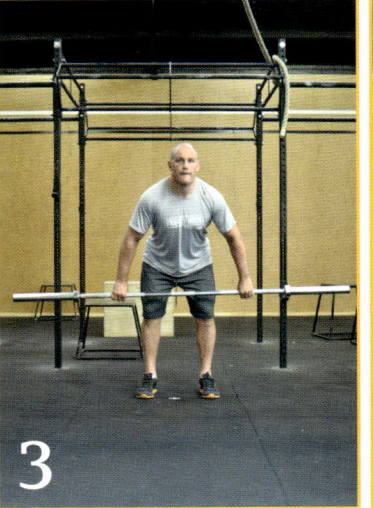
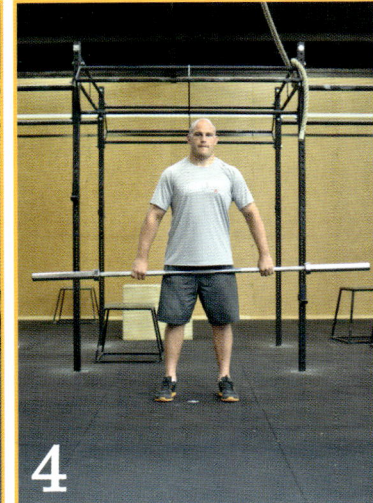

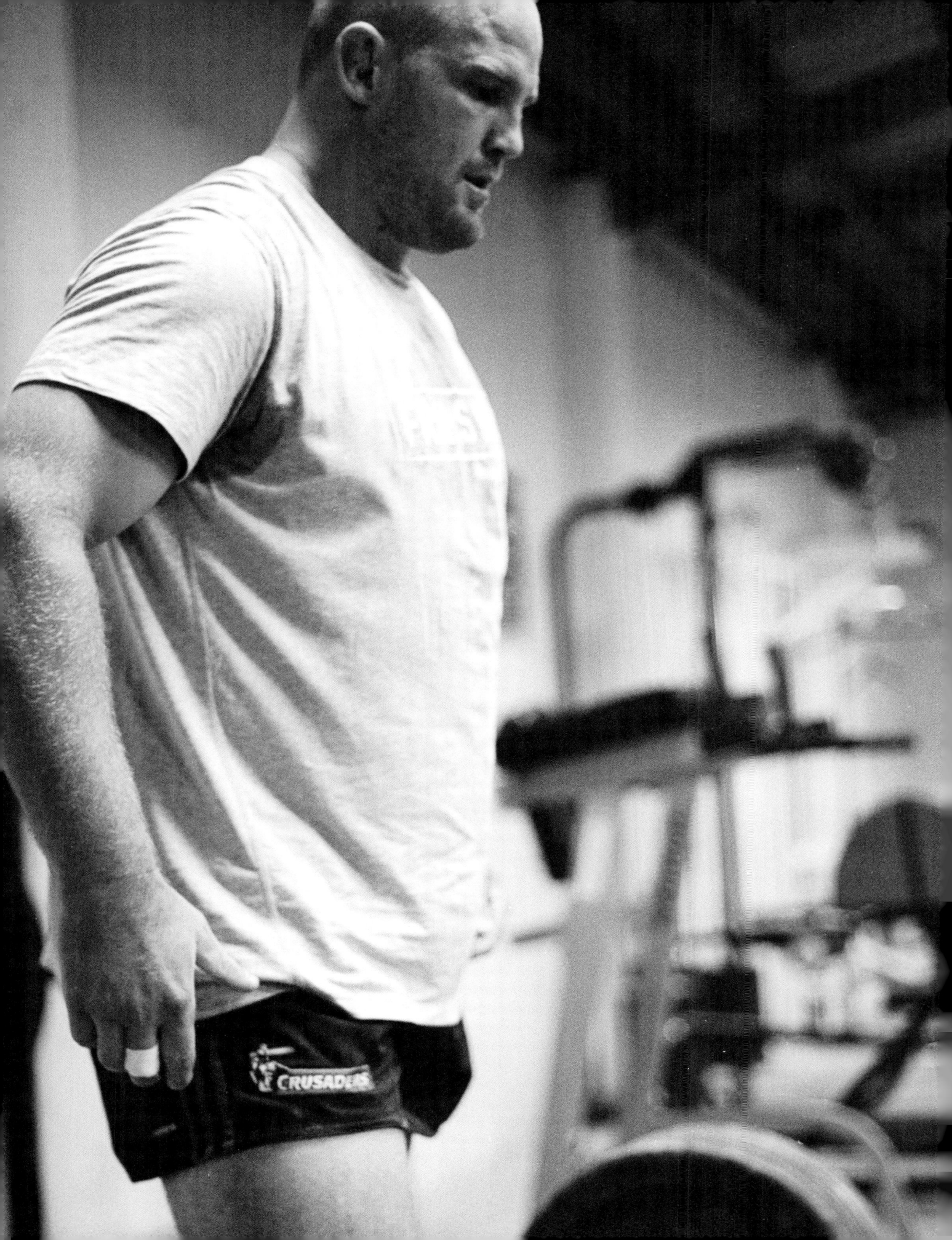

Dumbbell row

The dumbbell row is a great exercise to develop the major muscles in the back. The row movement can be performed standing or with a barbell, but to start, use a suitable dumbbell weight (something you can comfortably lift 10 to 15 times before failing or breaking form). Find a bench, or box, and rest the opposite hand and knee on one side. Keep your back arched and your elbows close to your body when lifting the weight. Without swinging your body, lift the dumbbell by driving your elbows as high as they can go, then control the weight slowly down.

BEGINNER: Find a weight that you can lift no more than
12 reps, 3 sets.

INTERMEDIATE: Lift a heavier weight that you can only repeat
8 reps, 4 sets.

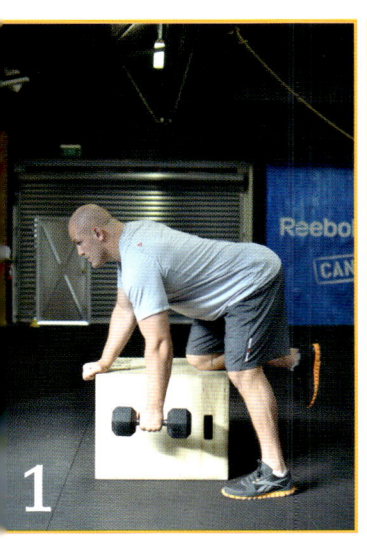
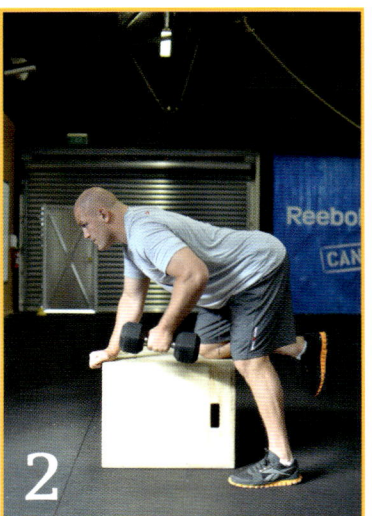
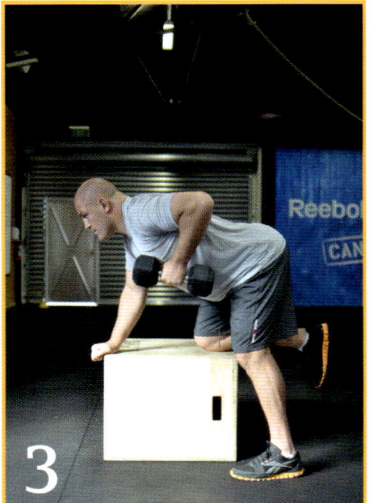
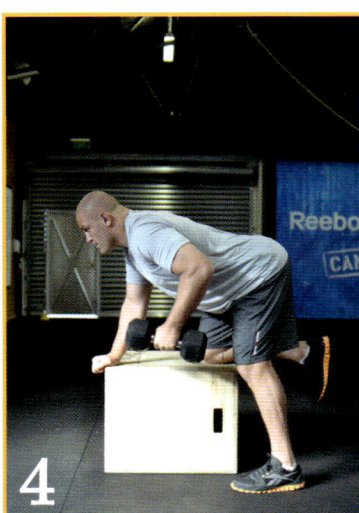

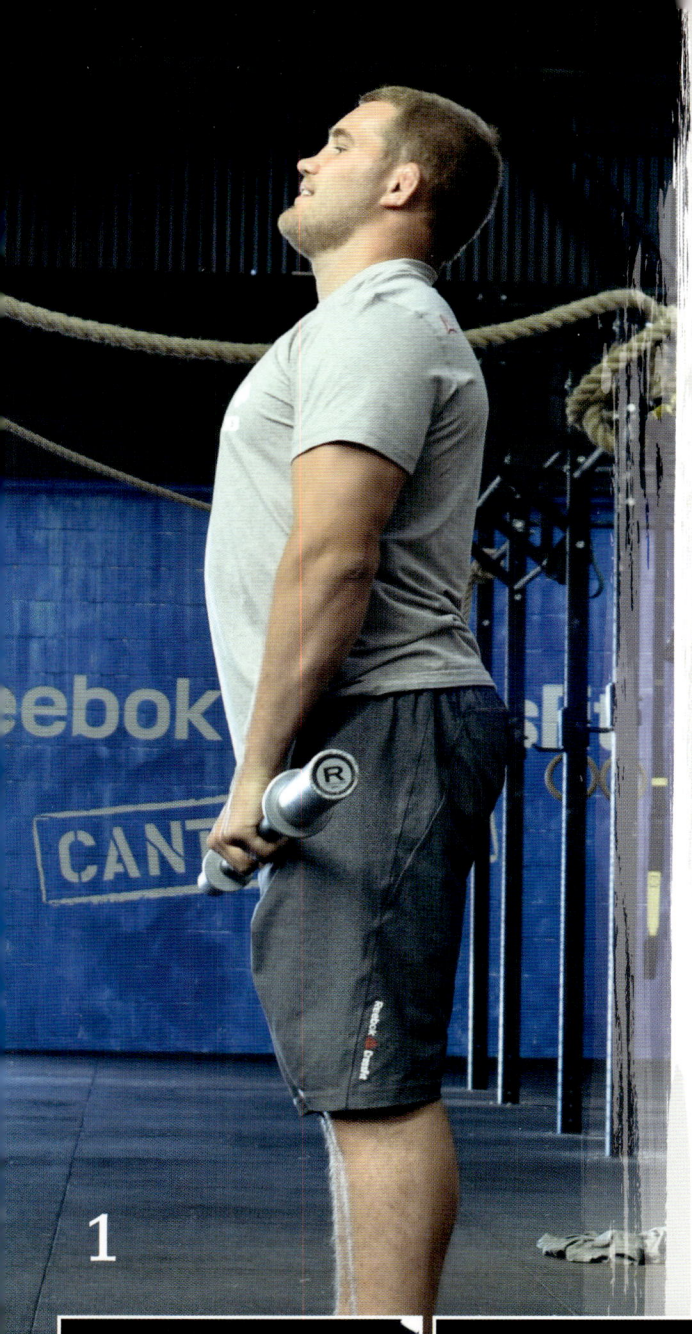

Upright row

This exercise focuses on developing the upper back, shoulders and arms. Hold the bar inside the width of the shoulder. Lift the bar to your chin, keeping it as close to your body as possible. Pause at the top. Then lower down the same path and repeat. Do this exercise at a controlled, steady pace.

BEGINNER: Find a weight that you can lift no more than 15 reps, 3 sets.

INTERMEDIATE: Lift a heavier weight that you can only repeat 10 reps, 4 sets.

1

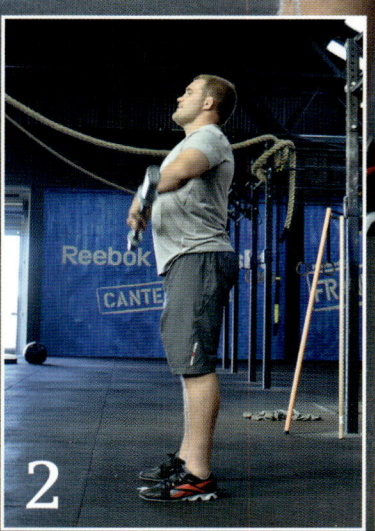

2

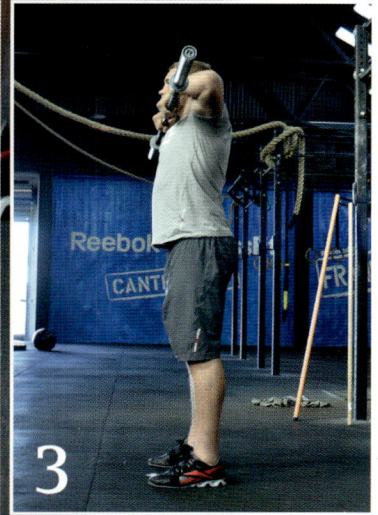

3

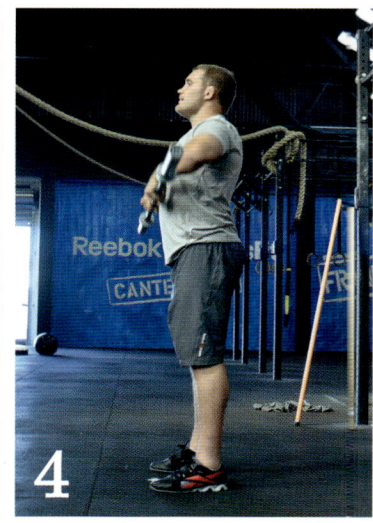

4

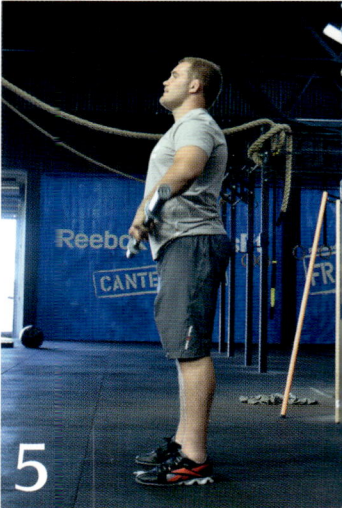

5

Shrugs

While the muscle groups in the upper back and shoulders don't appear to have a large range of movement, they can, however, grow to be immensely powerful. Learning to stand tall and shrug at the top of the clean or snatch movement is one of the keys to successfully coordinating your body's full power. Regularly practise this shrug movement during every snatch and clean session because it is the key to good powerlifting.

Set up the same way as you would for a clean or snatch, feet under the bar, shoulder width apart, knees bent, back straight with the chest up high. Start the lift by driving up through your heels and knees, then raise your body up by pushing your hips forward and shrugging your shoulders. Hold the shrug for a moment then return the bar back to the starting position and repeat.

BEGINNER: Find a weight that you can lift no more than
15 reps, 3 sets.

INTERMEDIATE: Lift a heavier weight that you can only repeat
10 reps, 4 sets.

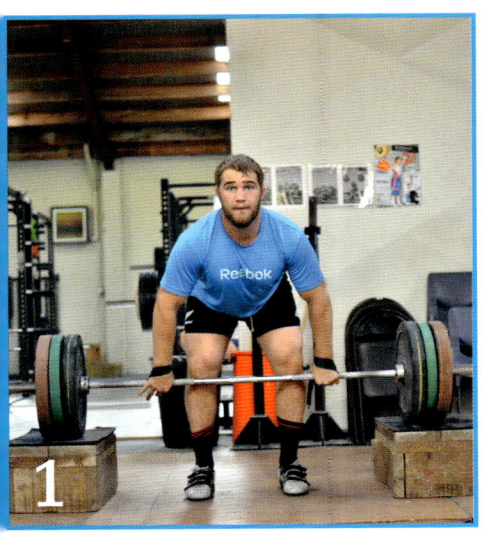 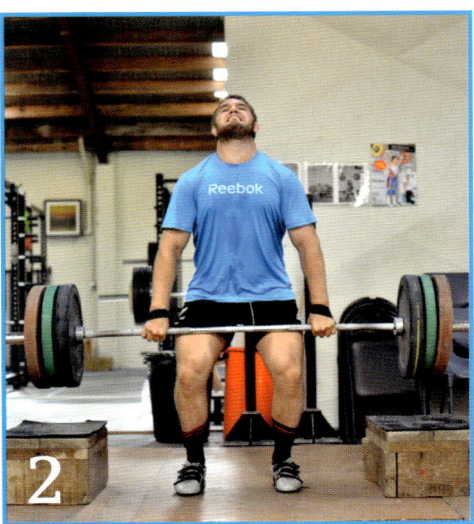 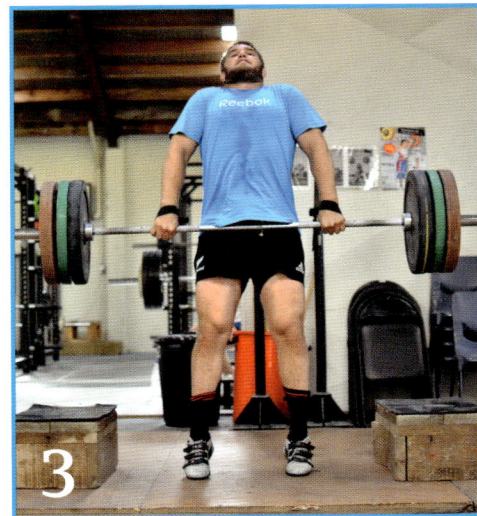

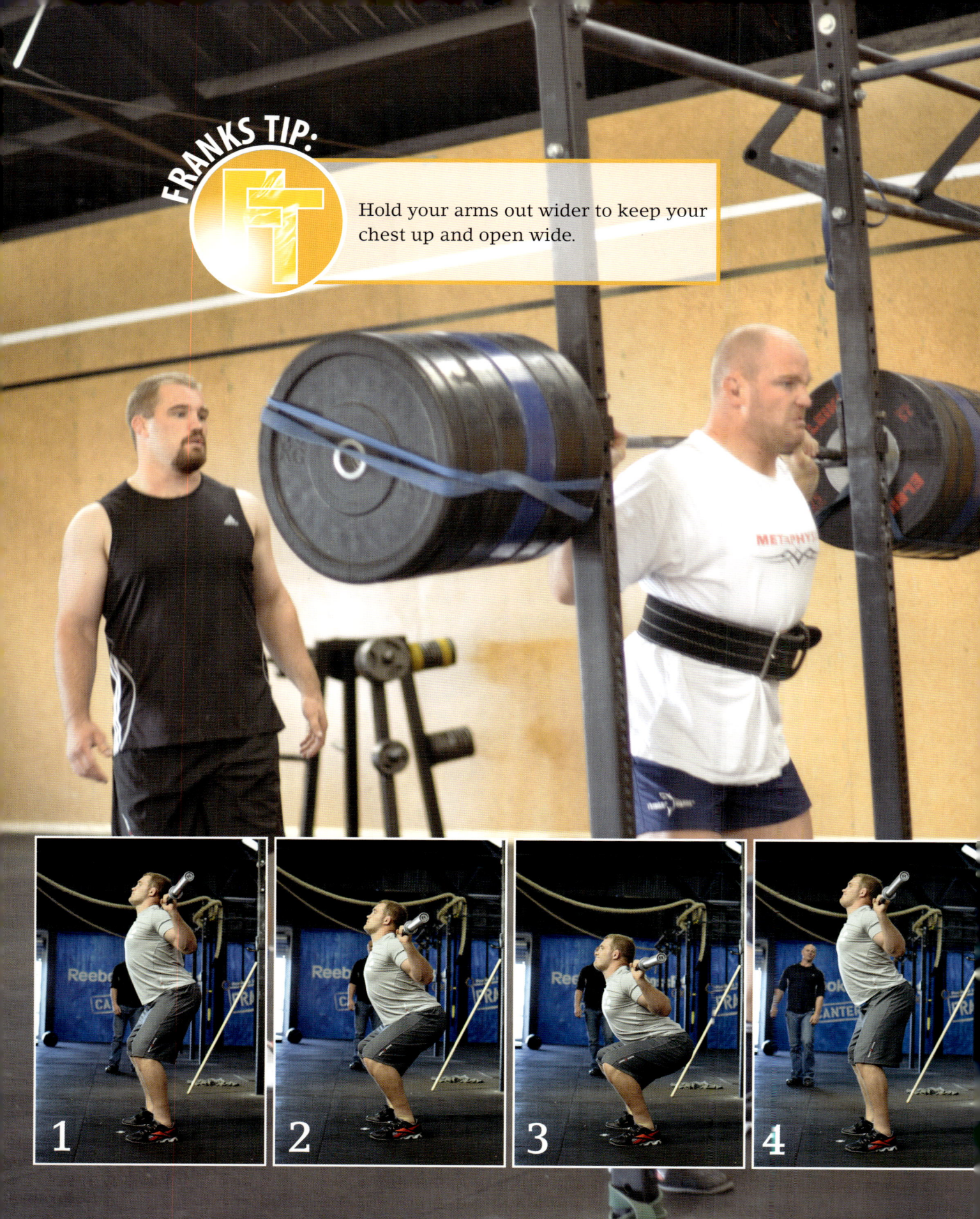

FRANKS TIP:

Hold your arms out wider to keep your chest up and open wide.

1

2

3

4

Back squat

The barbell back squat is an anchor exercise ideal for fast developing strength in the legs. Like all weighted exercises, form and posture are very important. Back squats can be done with much more weight than other weighted exercises (including the front squat), so to avoid long-term injury it is vital that care is taken to keep your back safe. If you are new to training, please use the bar only with no added weight to get used to lifting

At the gym you can use the weight rack or lifting cage to set the bar on before getting into position. Otherwise use the floor to set up the bar with a light weight then clean and jerk the weight up and over the shoulders before getting into a tall strong position, feet shoulder-width apart. Before each rep take a big breath in and hold it to tighten up the body's core.

Bend at the knees and hips, keeping your chest up as you lower into a deep squat. When coming back up focus both on keeping the back straight and pushing the knees outwards. Pushing the knees outward when lifting the weight up will help employ the powerful muscles in the back of your legs and bum. Finish the rep by standing up tall, taking another deep breath and repeating.

BEGINNER: Find a weight that you can lift no more than 15 reps, 3 sets.

INTERMEDIATE: Lift a heavier weight that you can only repeat 10 reps, 4 sets.

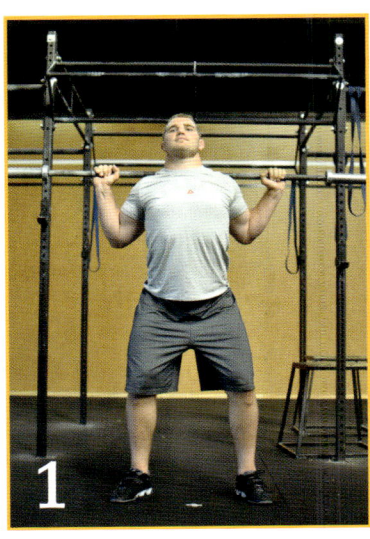
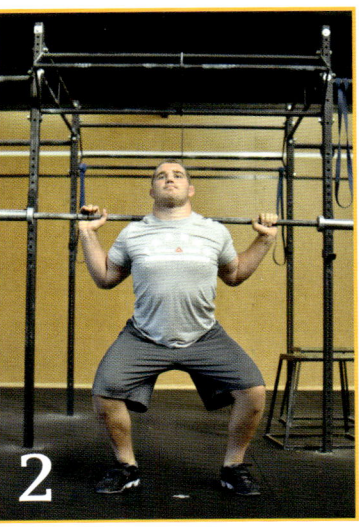
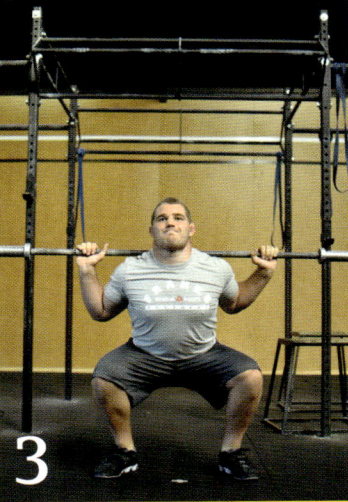
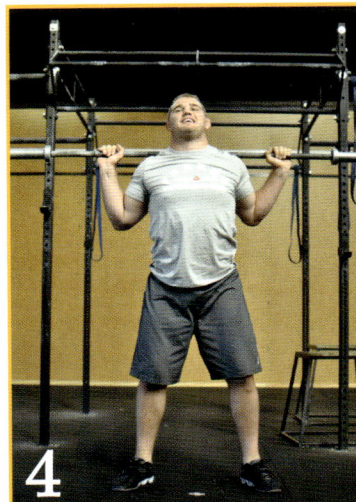

Calf raisers

Your feet are the foundation of your body. The calf muscles in your legs control the movement of your feet, so needless to say keeping them strong is vital to basic movements like running and jumping. Increasing the strength of your calf muscles will provide a better platform for the rest of your body, improve balance, and create a more explosive step.

Using only your body weight find a step or plate and hang one of your heels over the edge. With your opposite leg off the ground, lower your heel down to the ground then lift high to your toes. Intermediate athletes can hold additional weight to increase the loading on the calf muscles.

BEGINNER: 15 reps each leg, 3 sets.

INTERMEDIATE: 10 reps each leg, 4 sets, holding extra weight that you can repeat.

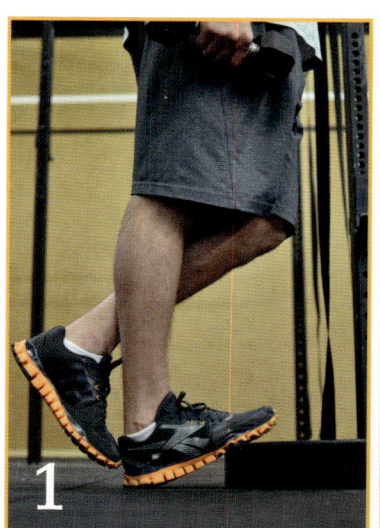
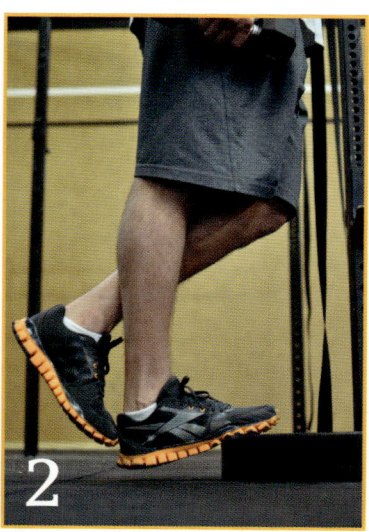
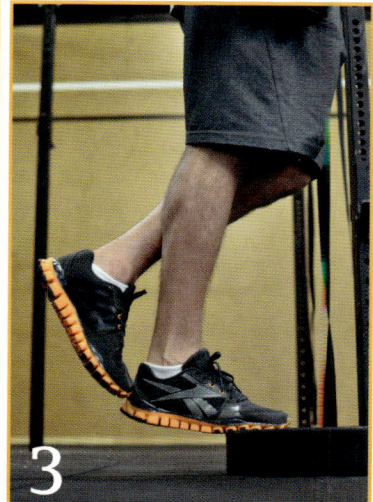
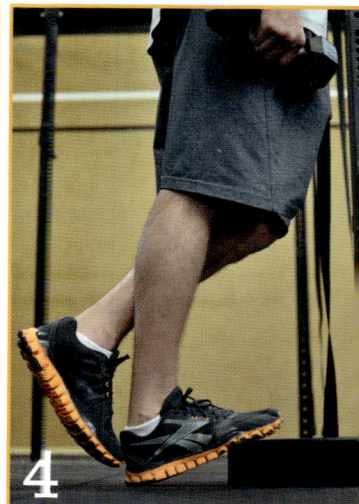

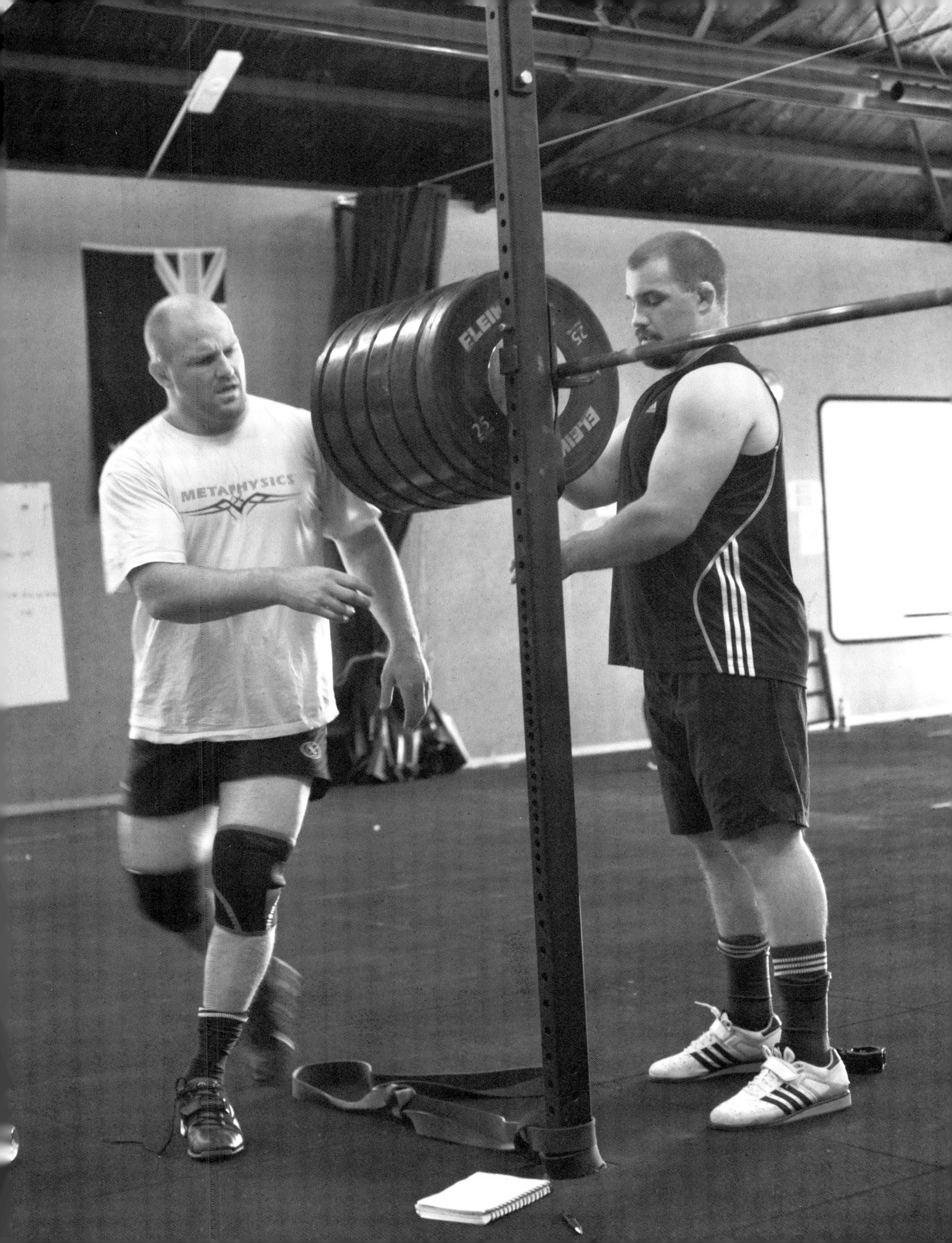

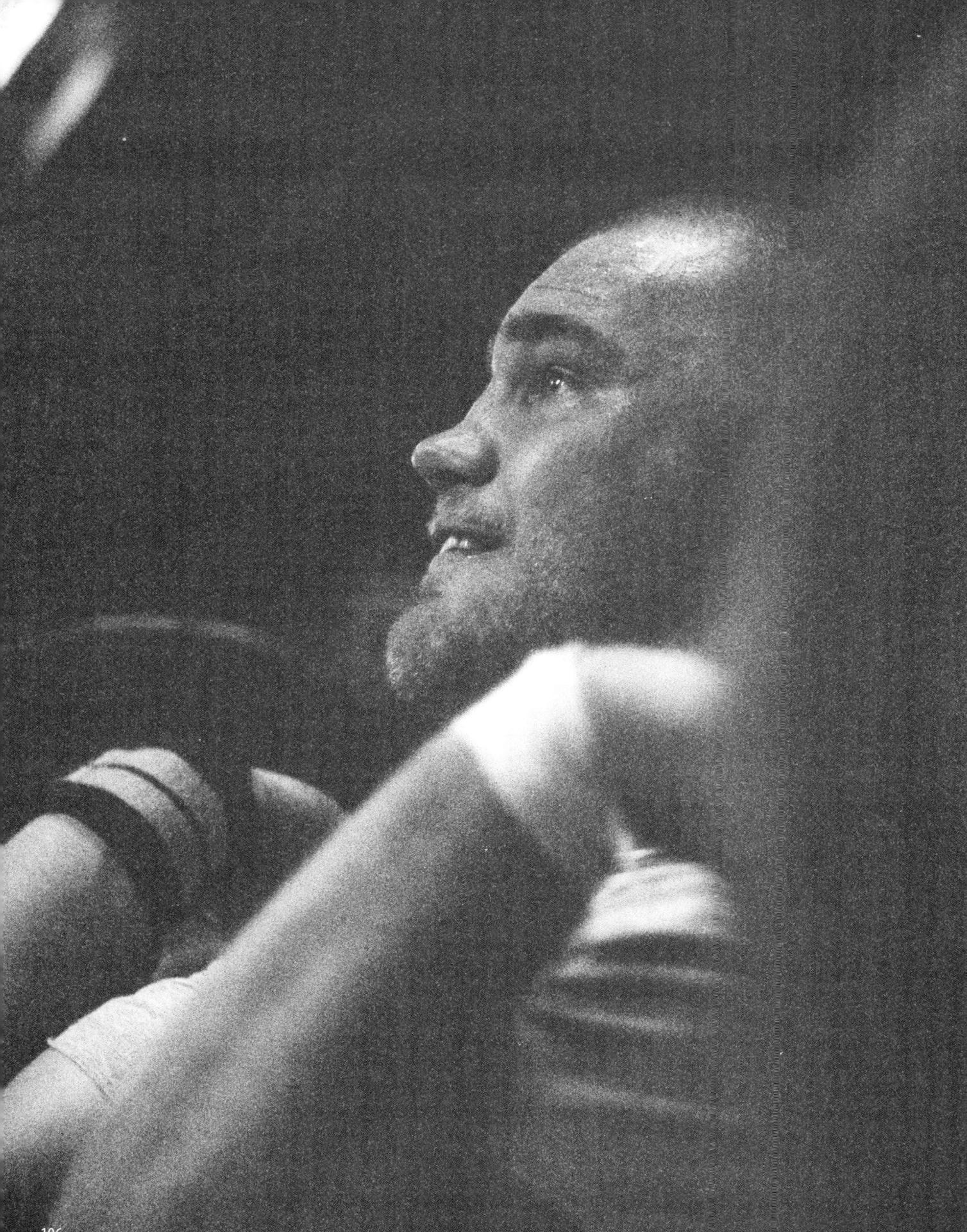

OLYMPIC WEIGHTLIFTING EXERCISES

(featured in order of the

Olympic Weightlifting Power Program)

Put simply, Olympic weightlifting is about placing your body between the weight and the ground: cleaning weight from off the ground, jerking or snatching it above your head. These are the fundamentals of manufacturing a stronger body. Not only do your muscles get stronger, but so do your ligaments and tendons, not to mention your mind and overall muscle coordination.

Olympic movements can be complicated, and if done wrongly can compromise an athlete's body. It is recommended to start with a wooden staff/broomstick or a barbell with no weight. Ideally, a coach is present to give you verbal feedback on posture improvements and muscle firing order. To avoid back injuries when lifting weights, make sure you always engage your core muscles by taking a deep breath and holding before each lift.

The hook grip will need to be practised from the start. This grip will better lock your hands to the bar. The grip is not very comfortable to start with but you will get used to it over time, and will really need it once heavy lifts are performed.

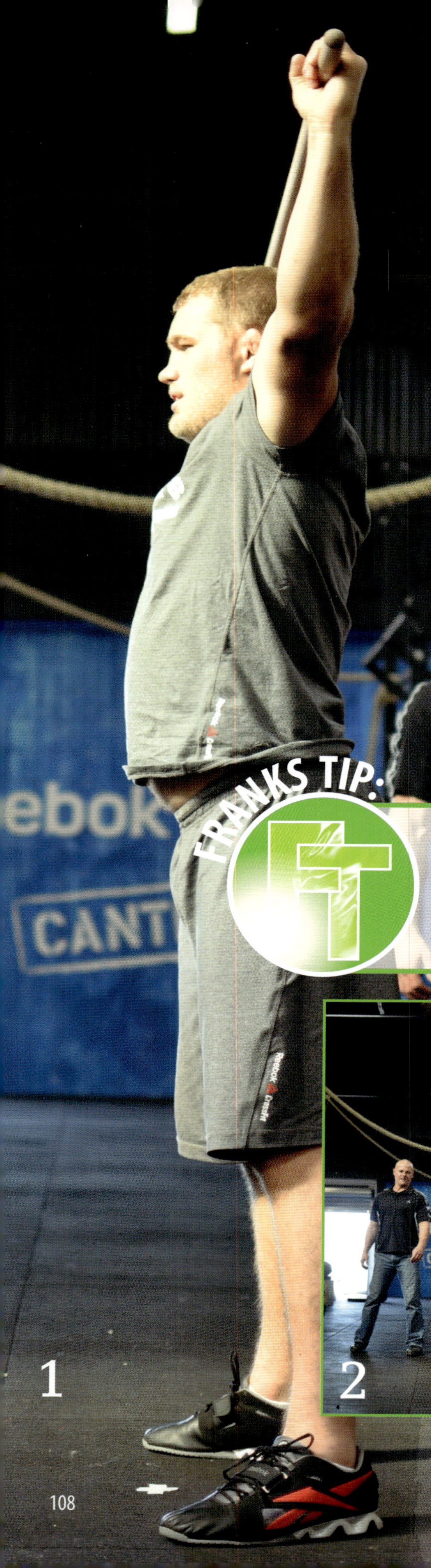

Snatch squat

Otherwise known as the overhead squat, without good shoulder and hip flexibility this exercise can take time to master. For beginners, start with a stick or bar (with no weight) resting across the back of the shoulders, hands wide apart, feet slightly wider than shoulder-width apart, weight on your heels and toes pointing away from each other. Lift the bar above your head, locking your arms out to full extension, and continue to actively push the bar upwards for the entire duration of the exercise.

BEGINNER: 5 sets of 5 repetitions with an easy weight.

INTERMEDIATE: 5 sets of 3 repetitions with a heavier, harder weight.

FRANKS TIP:

If you are having trouble getting into position, try a slightly wider stance. If you cannot lower into a deep squat without compromising your form, just go down as far as you can before your chest and head dip forward.

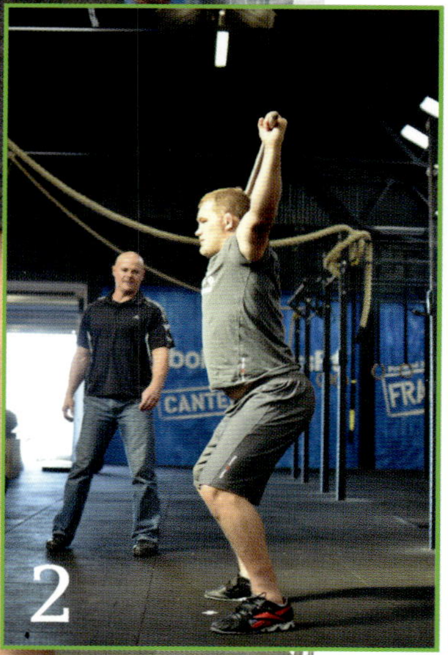

1

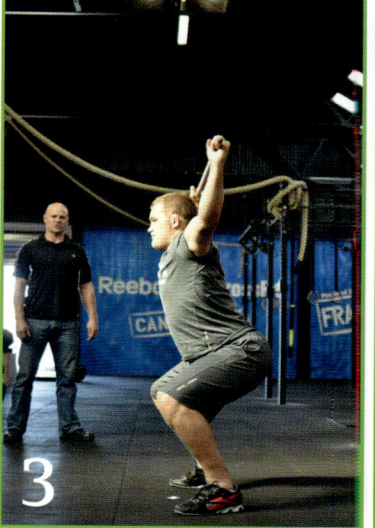

2

3

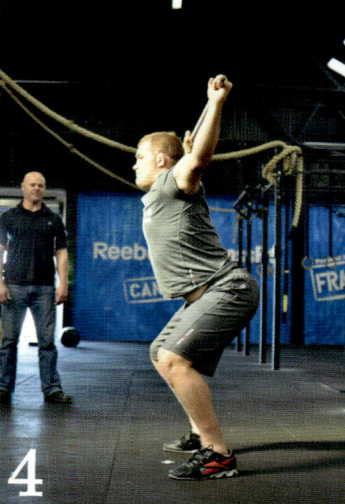

4

Drop snatch

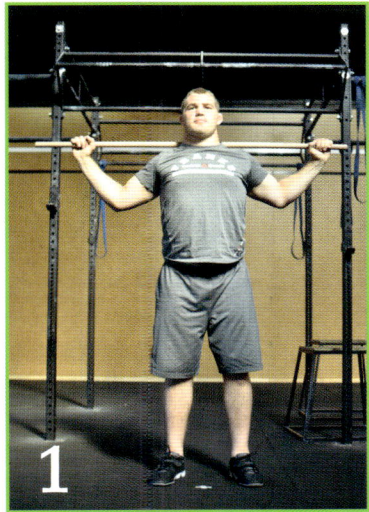

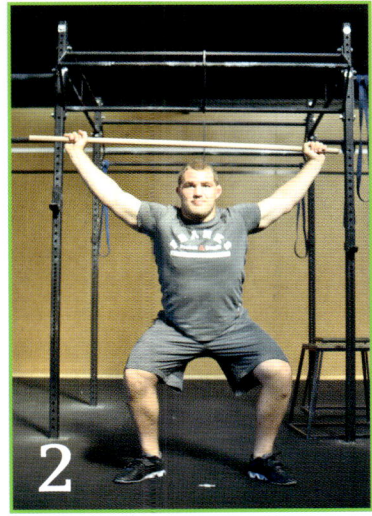

Speed cannot be emphasised enough when performing the drop snatch. Even when learning the movement with only a light weight it is important to practise the same technique as if you were lifting a lot of weight. Start the movement with the bar across the back of your shoulders, hands spread wide and feet starting shoulder-width apart. Take a deep breath and stand tall. Bounce the weight slightly upwards before sliding your feet out, dropping into a full squat. Imagine yourself pushing your body downwards with your arms against the bar. This movement is an art. If you are not part of a lifting club and don't have a trainer to help you with your posture and technique, study as many credible video references as you can find online.

BEGINNER: 5 sets of 5 repetitions with an easy weight.

INTERMEDIATE: 5 sets of 3 repetitions with a heavier, harder weight.

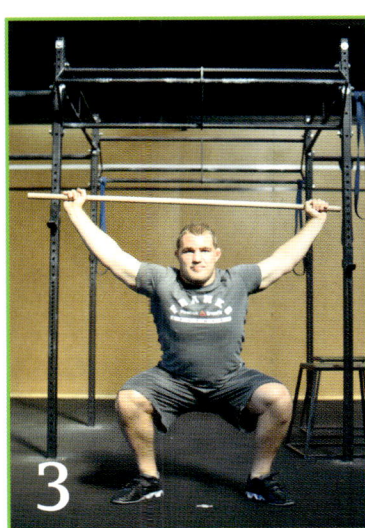

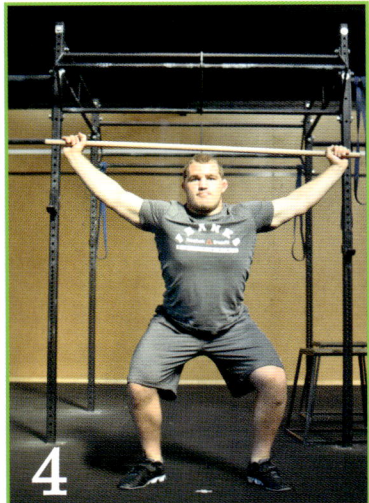

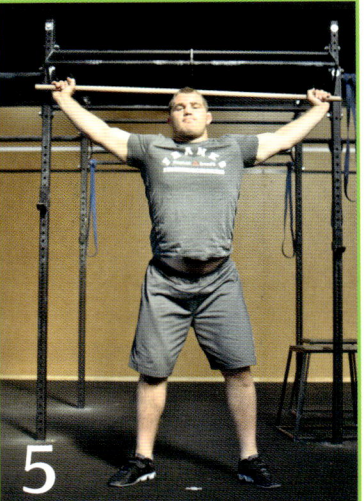

Snatch from waist

Because of the upright starting position, the snatch from waist exercise is more explosive than the hang or floor pull. Start the movement by standing up straight with a wide hook grip across the bar. Dip and shrug the weight violently to generate enough upward momentum on the bar to quickly pull yourself under it, into an overhead squat position. Keeping the chest up, drive through the heels to stand the bar up over your head, keeping the arms actively pressing upwards.

BEGINNER: 5 sets of 5 repetitions with an easy weight.

INTERMEDIATE: 5 sets of 3 repetitions with a heavier, harder weight.

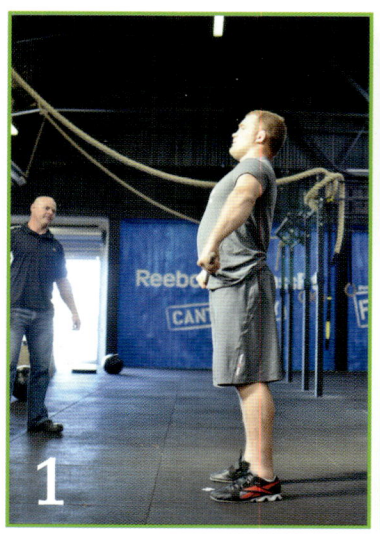
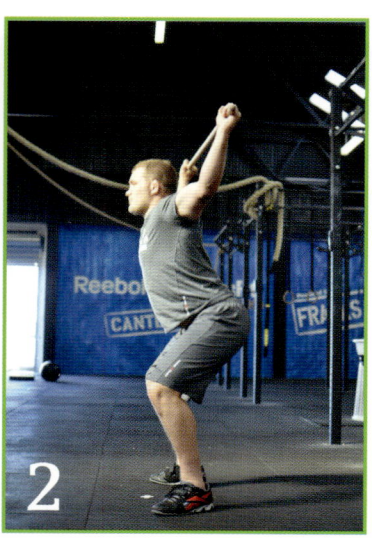
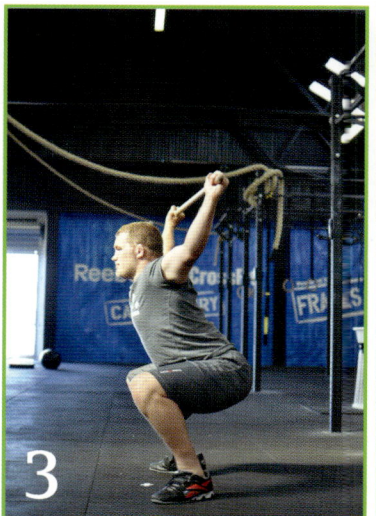
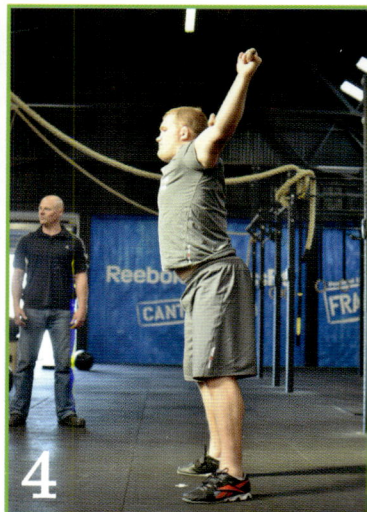

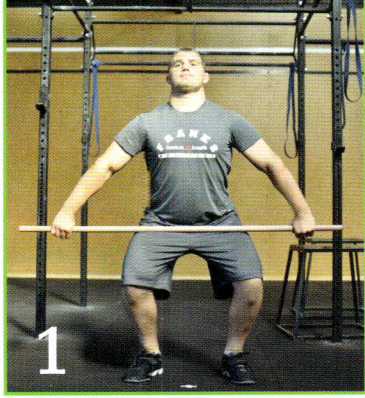

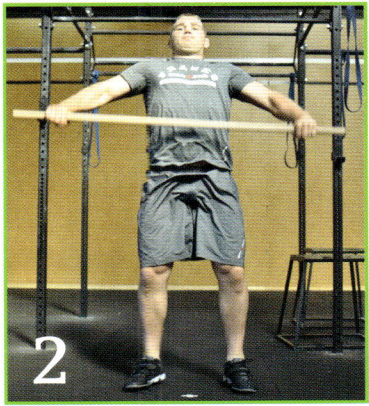

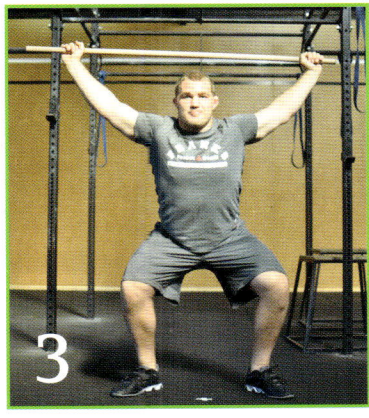

Snatch from hang

The hang snatch is the same movement as the snatch from waist except you get more run-in and more opportunity to swing your hips forward and shrug the bar upward. Bend at the knees and let the bar slide down your leg to the mid-thigh position. Quickly stand straight up on your heels by emphasising the swinging of your hips and shrugging your shoulders upwards. Your body and shoulders should do all of the work, not your arms. When fully upright, dive under the weight by quickly sliding your feet out and fully bending at the knees. Use your arms to push your body under the bar, pushing your head through so your hands feel almost behind you. Finish the lift by standing up.

BEGINNER: 5 sets of 5 repetitions with an easy weight.

INTERMEDIATE: 5 sets of 3 repetitions with a heavier, harder weight.

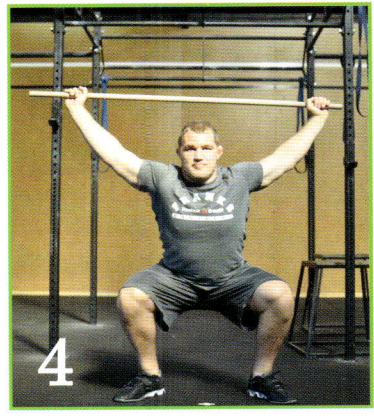

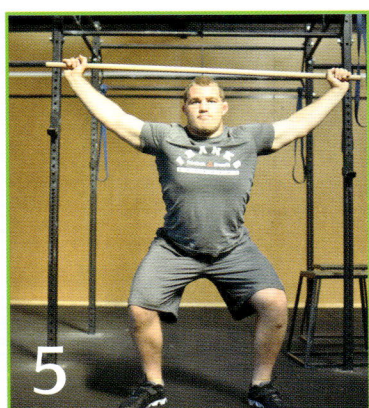

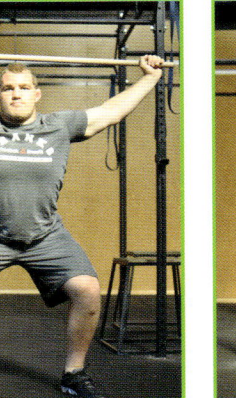

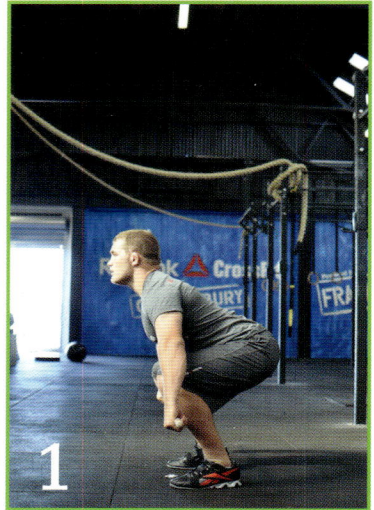

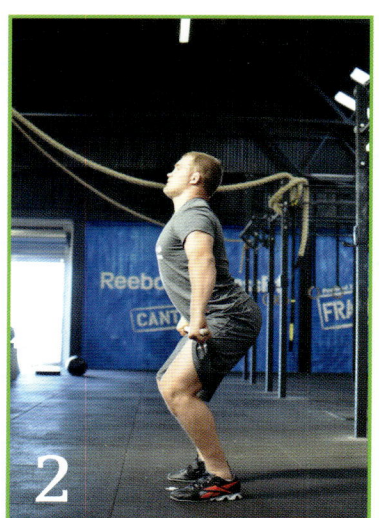

Snatch pull

The key to any snatch lift is to generate as much power from the strongest muscle groups in the body, sending the barbell upwards. For beginners, there is a temptation to use your arms to snatch the bar above your head, but this is a rookie mistake. The legs, hips, and shrug of the back and shoulders should generate enough upward force to only just need muscles in the arms to pull yourself under the bar and quickly into position. Practising the snatch pull will help coordinate the first phases of that movement.

The snatch pull will improve overall power and strength but most importantly help perfect the firing order of the various muscle groups in your body. Start in the power snatch position. Go through the same initial series of movements as the full snatch, only stopping to hold on the final shrug phase.

BEGINNER: 5 sets of 5 repetitions with an easy weight.

INTERMEDIATE: 5 sets of 3 repetitions with a heavier, harder weight.

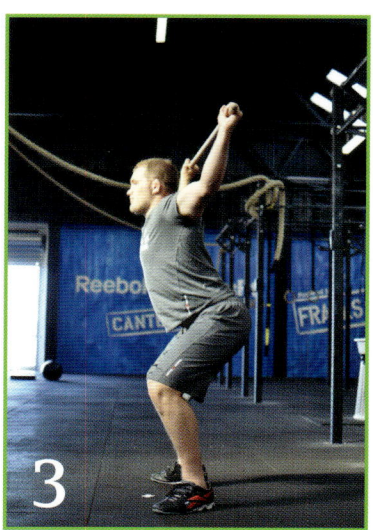

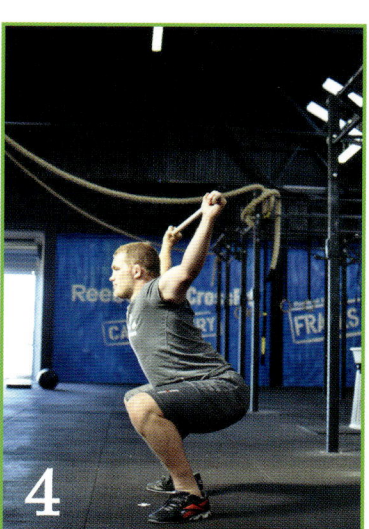

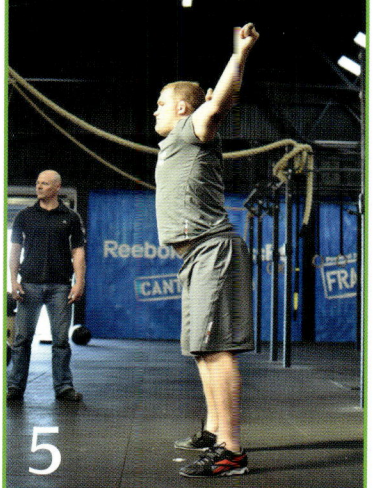

Power snatch from floor

Snatching a bar from the floor position allows a larger range of movement than the waist or hang snatch, but the start of the lift is actually quite slow. It is not until the bar is above the knees that the lift needs to become aggressive. Set up with feet shoulder-width apart. Bend deep at the knees like you are about to jump up high (backside not up high in the air) and take a wide grip of the bar (or stick). Keeping the bar as close to the body as possible, slowly pull it back through the heels until it reaches above the knee. Then repeat the same movement as the snatch from hang above.

BEGINNER: 5 sets of 5 repetitions with an easy weight.

INTERMEDIATE: 5 sets of 3 repetitions with a heavier, harder weight.

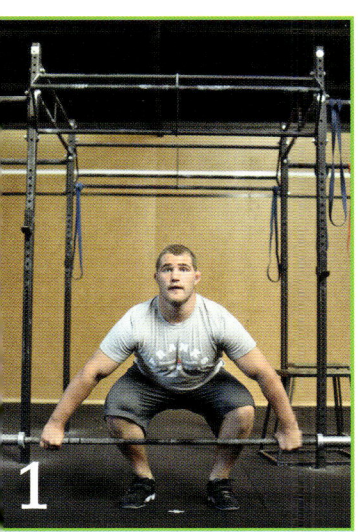
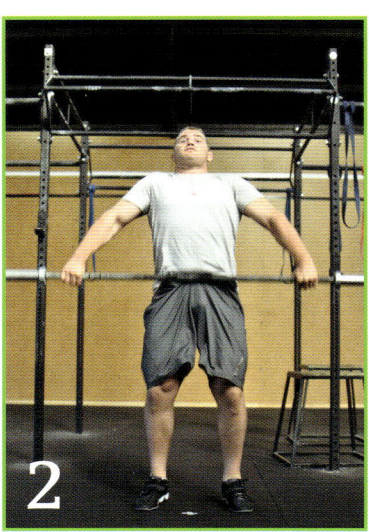
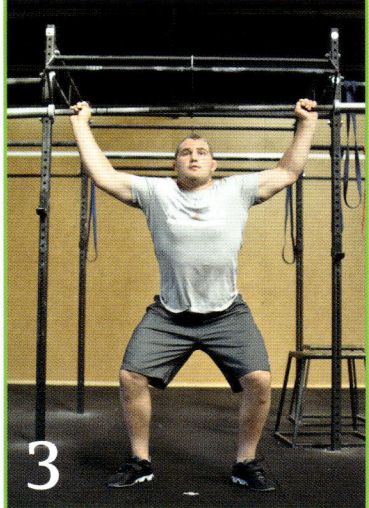
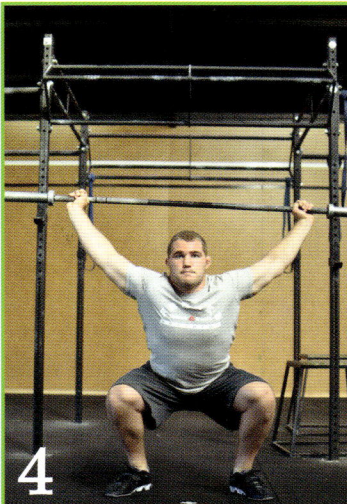

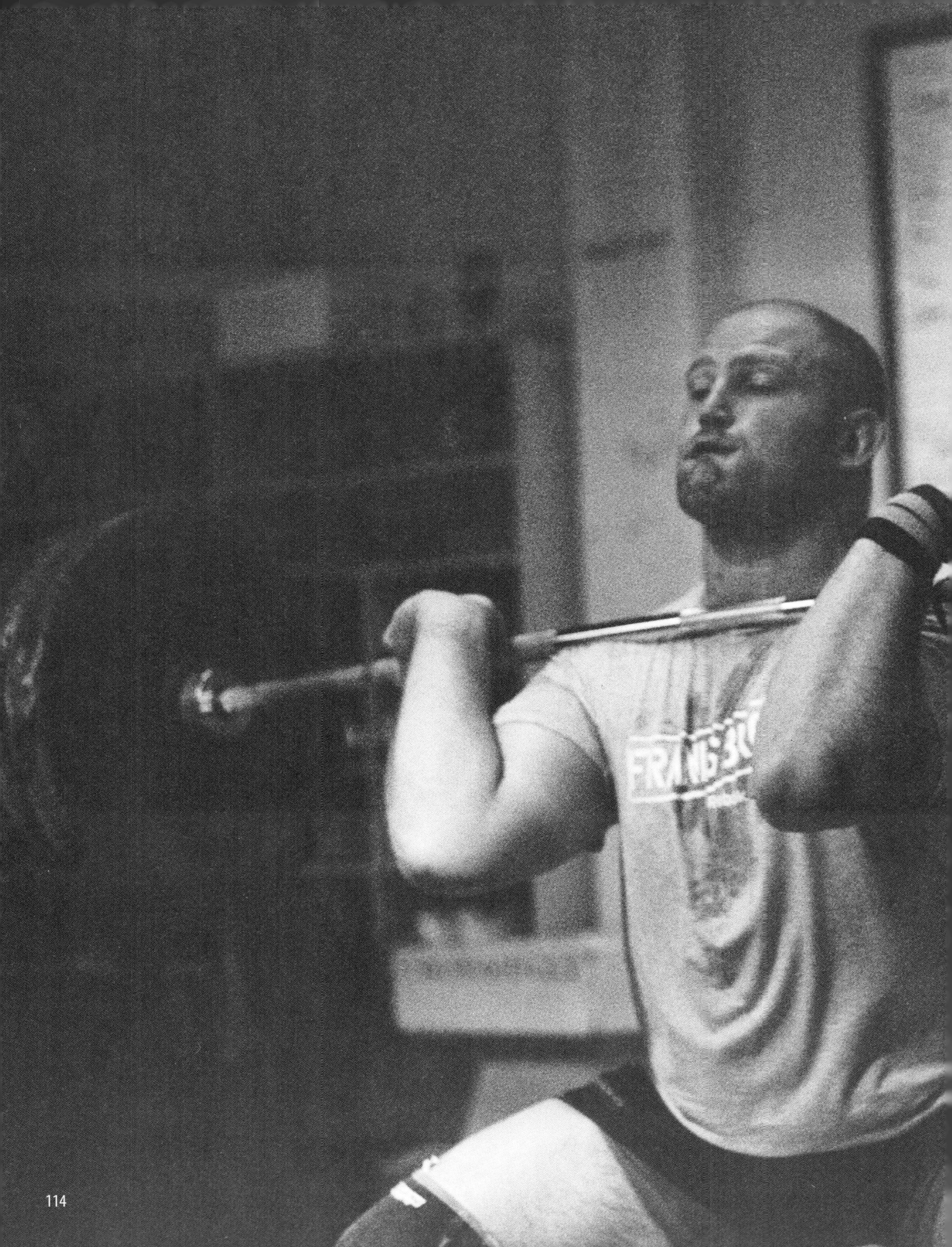

Cleans

Olympic lifting coach Lee Attrill will tell you the clean movement is the basis of the Franks brothers' strength and power. The fundamental movement involves efficiently lifting a weight from the floor, hang, or waist, up to a 'racked position' across the front of the shoulders with the elbows pointing through. This movement is one of the most common exercises found in the Franks routine and is excellent for developing full body power and strength.

Watching Ben and Owen go through 5 set of 3 reps makes it look too easy.

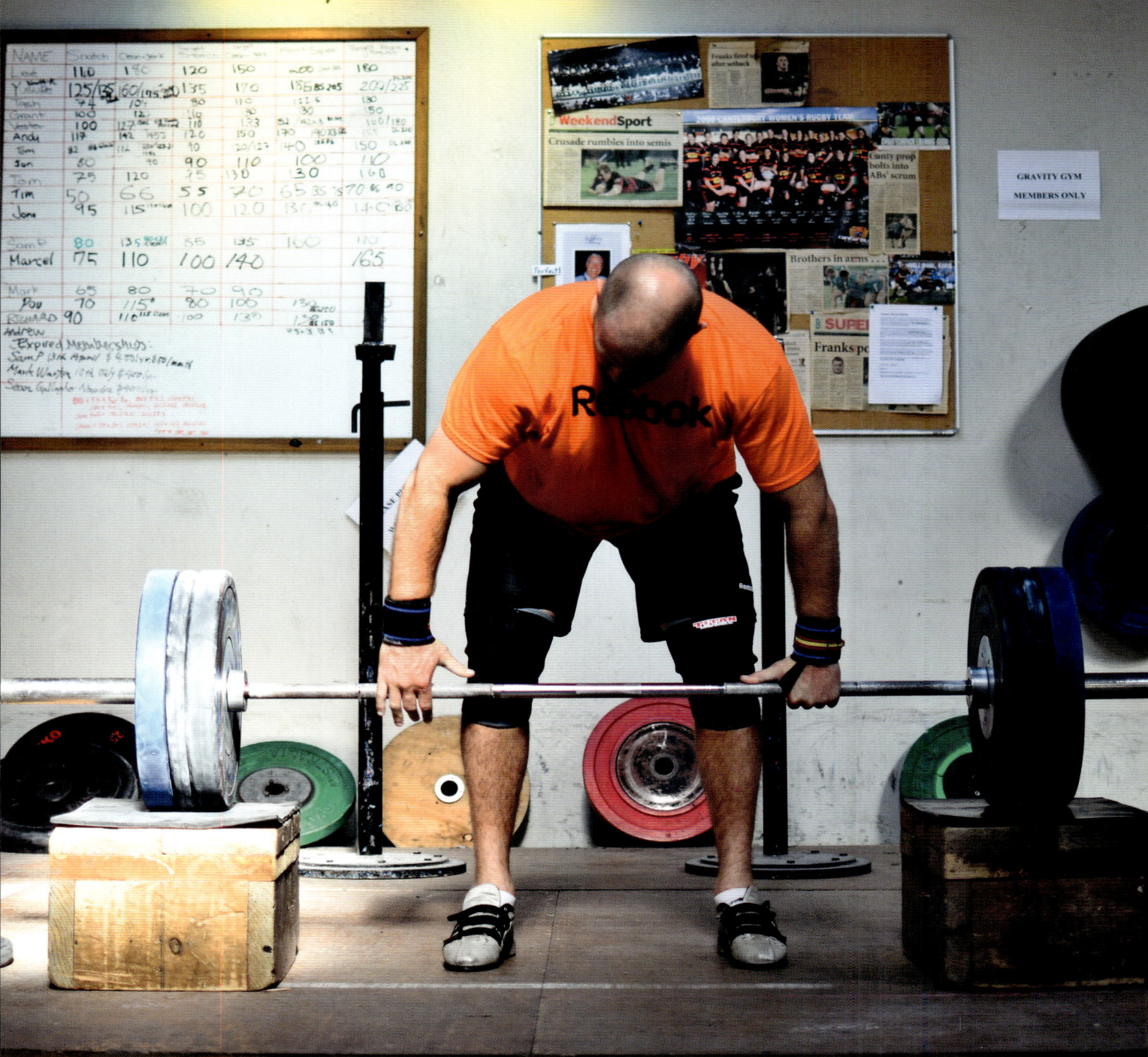

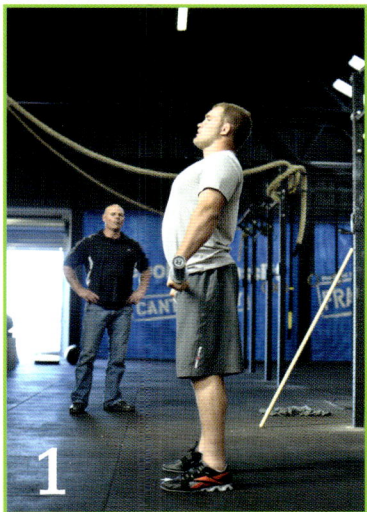

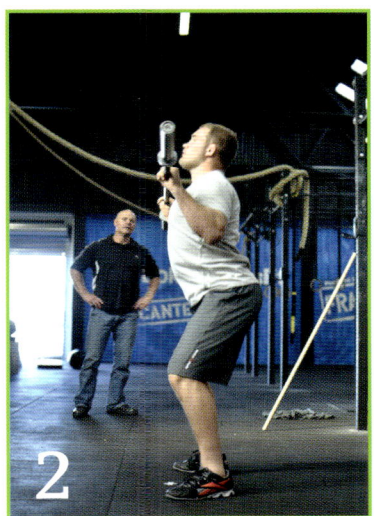

Clean from waist

Because the bar has little chance to gain momentum, start with a lighter weight or just the bar, hands shoulder-width apart in a hook grip with the body standing straight up, and clean. Dip and shrug from your shoulders, pull your elbows to the sky, and quickly dive under the bar by bending the knees and sliding the feet slightly wider. Catch the weight across the front of the shoulders and lift it to a standing position. Then lower the weight back to the waist and repeat.

BEGINNER: 5 sets of 5 repetitions with an easy weight.

INTERMEDIATE: 5 sets of 3 repetitions with a heavier, harder weight.

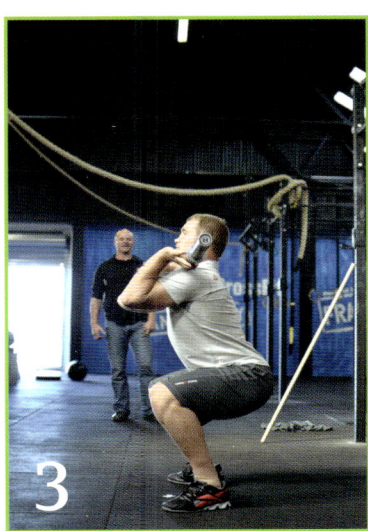

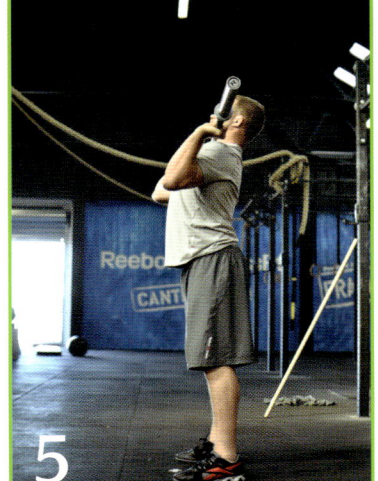

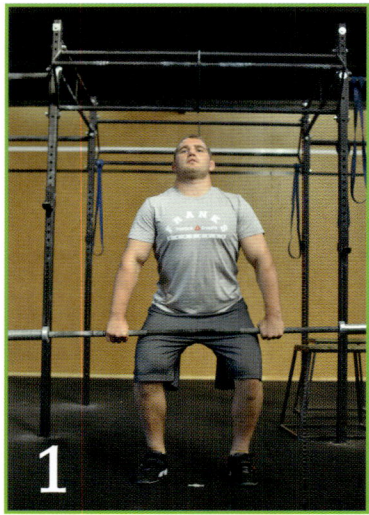

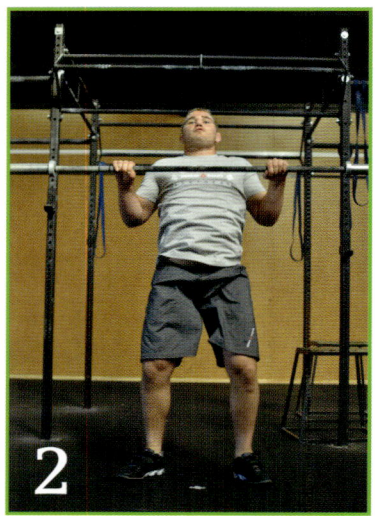

Clean from hang

Once you are set with the bar hanging mid-thighs, weight on your heels, chest up, emphasise the swing forward of your hips, quickly followed by the upward shrug of the shoulders to send the bar upwards allowing your body to drop underneath the weight, getting your elbows through. Finish by standing straight up with the weight racked across the front of the shoulders.

BEGINNER: 5 sets of 5 repetitions with an easy weight.

INTERMEDIATE: 5 sets of 3 repetitions with a heavier, harder weight.

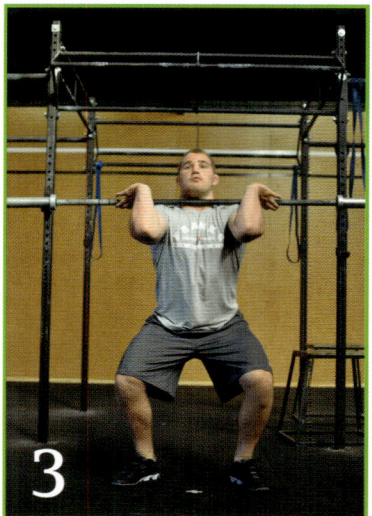

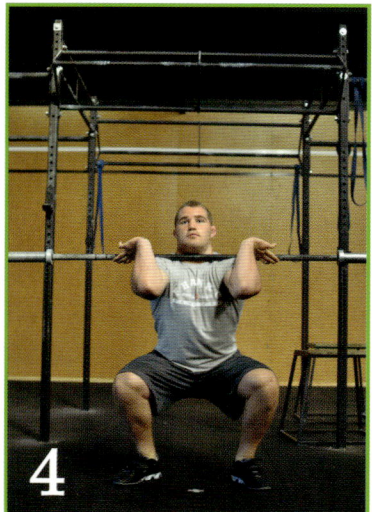

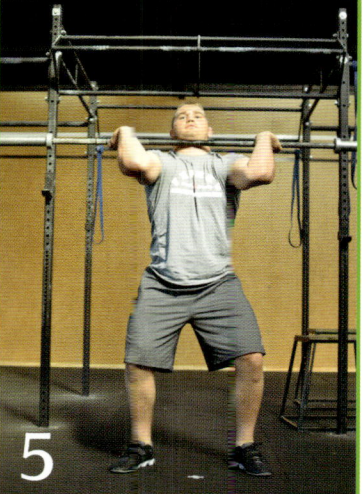

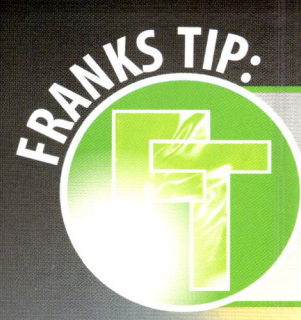

FRANKS TIP:

As you shrug and drop under the bar, concentrate on leading your elbows 'through and high' as you drop into position. When standing the weight up, there is a tendency to lean forward, so imagine lifting tall from your elbows to keep your chest up.

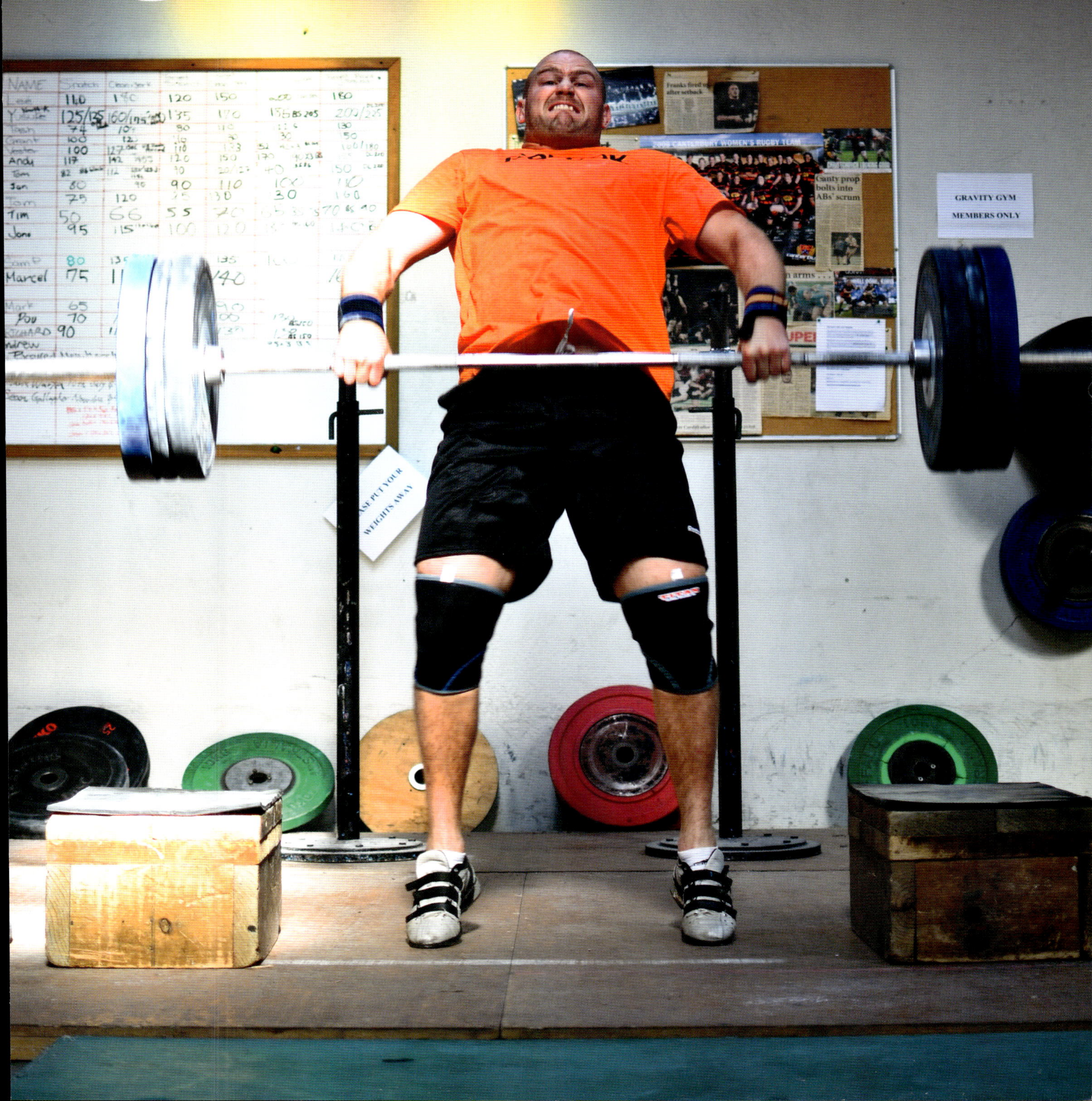

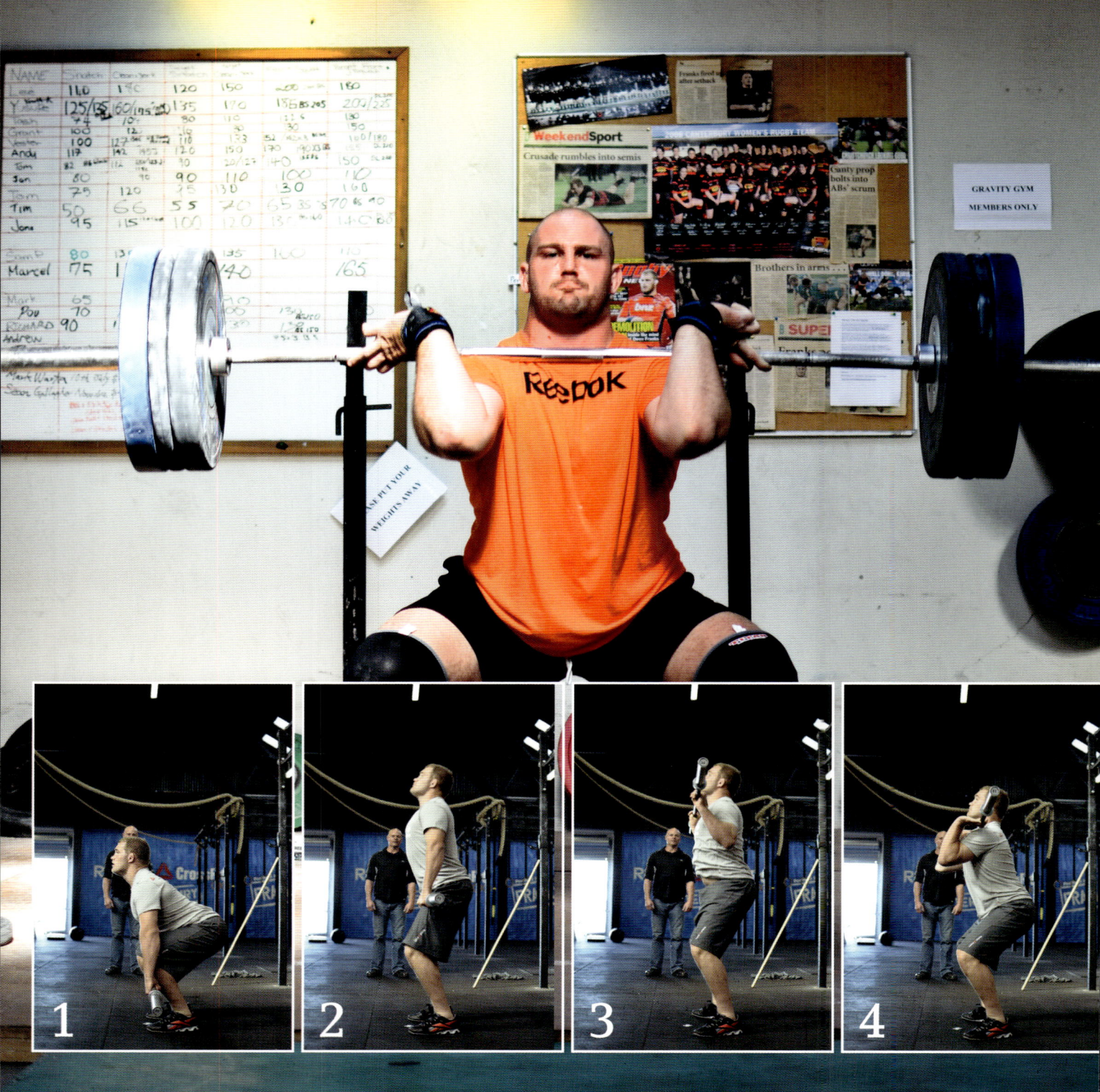

Clean from floor

Cleaning a solid weight from the floor is going to make you stronger. Adding this exercise to your program will add explosive power to your entire body. Start with your shoelaces directly under the bar, hands shoulder-width apart, knees bent in a position like you are about to leap straight up in the air. With your weight on your heels, keep your chest up as you smoothly raise the bar above the knees. Then explode the hips forward and shrug the shoulders upwards into an upright position before diving under the bar, pulling your elbows through. Lift upwards, thinking 'elbows first' as you lift the weight to a fully standing position. As simple as this movement sounds, perfecting it takes a lot of practice. When beginning to learn the clean don't be a hero, keep the weight light until you master a safe technique.

BEGINNER: 5 sets of 5 repetitions with an easy weight.

INTERMEDIATE: 5 sets of 3 repetitions with a heavier, harder weight.

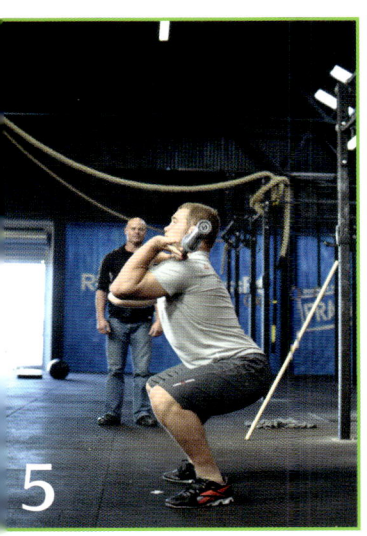
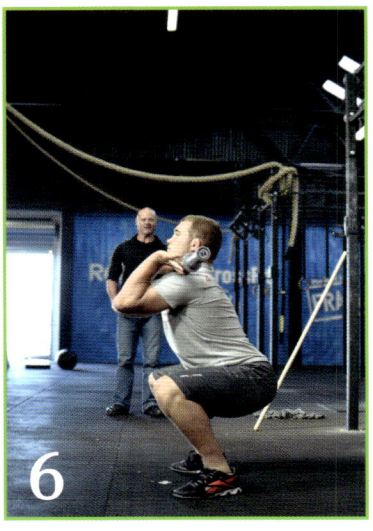
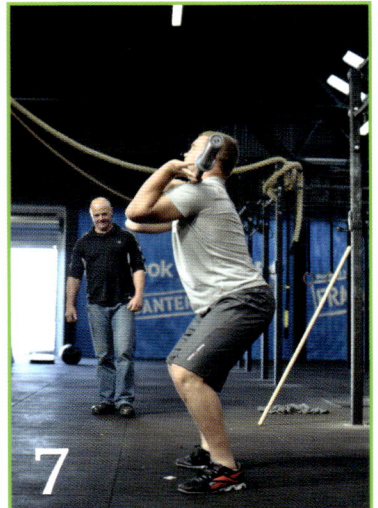
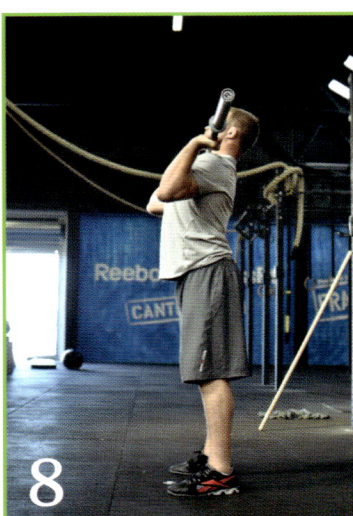

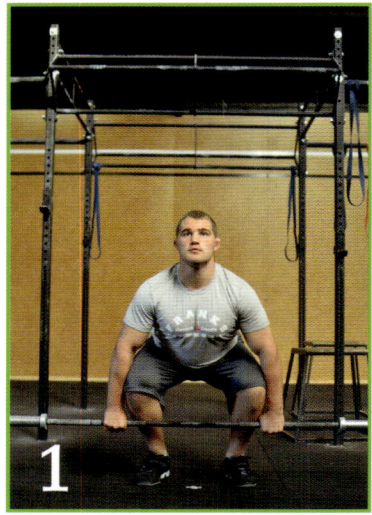

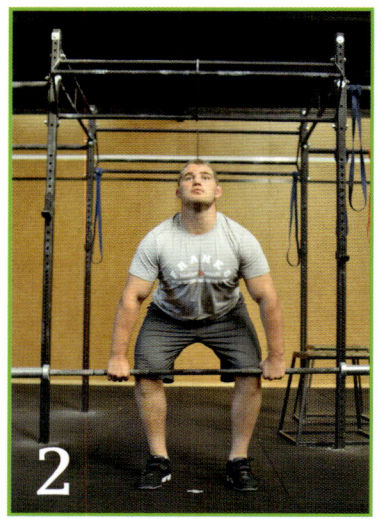

Clean pull

A great exercise in their own right, the clean pulls are also an excellent movement to practise the most explosive part of the clean's shrug movement. Power through the heels and coordinate the big shrug by rocking onto your toes. The bar stays close to the body throughout the movement and finishes at waist hip height. Good form is important, so if you don't have a trainer who can check your technique, why not do what the pros do and set up a video camera to study and critique?

BEGINNER: 5 sets of 5 repetitions with an easy weight.

INTERMEDIATE: 5 sets of 3 repetitions with a heavier, harder weight.

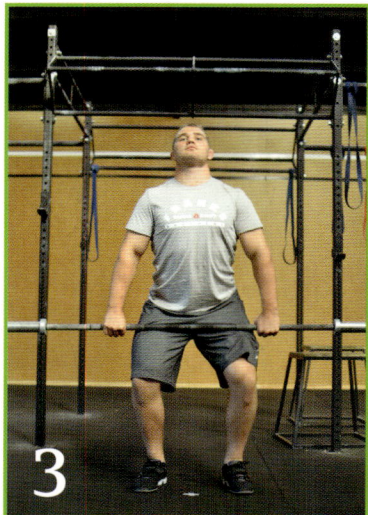

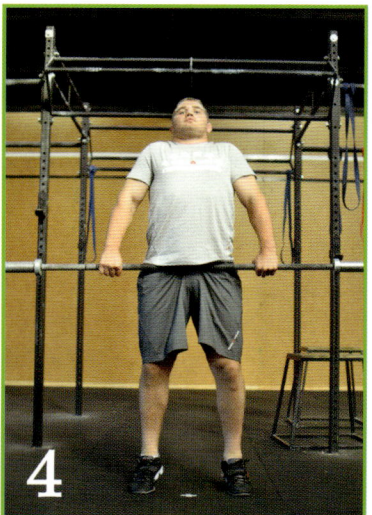

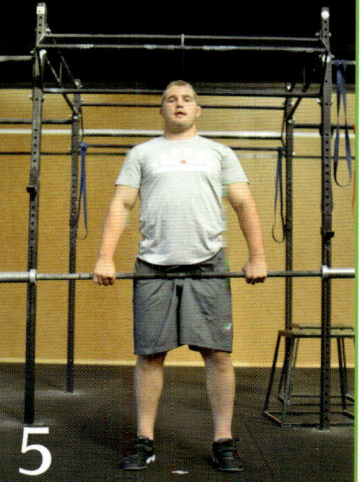

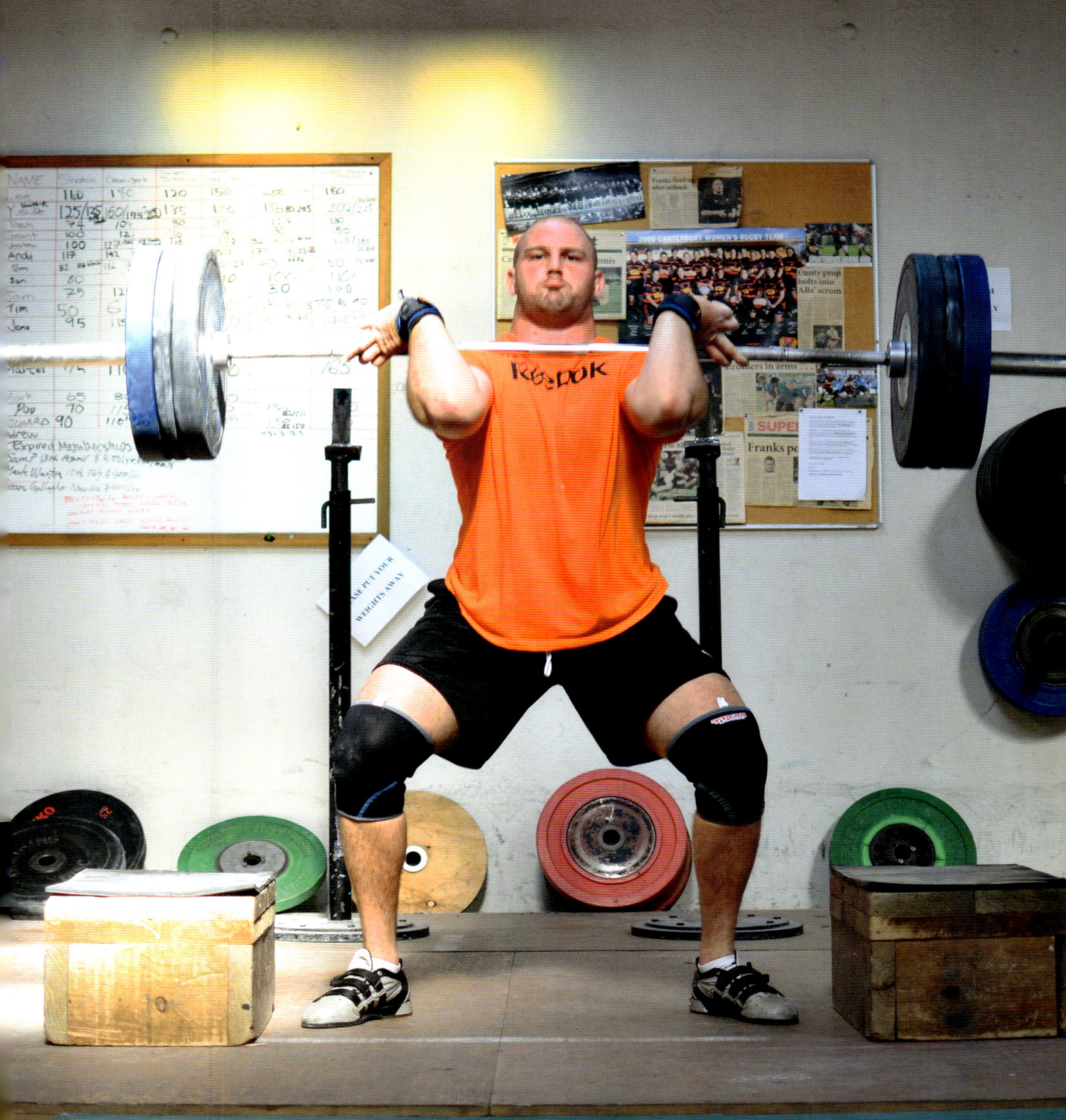

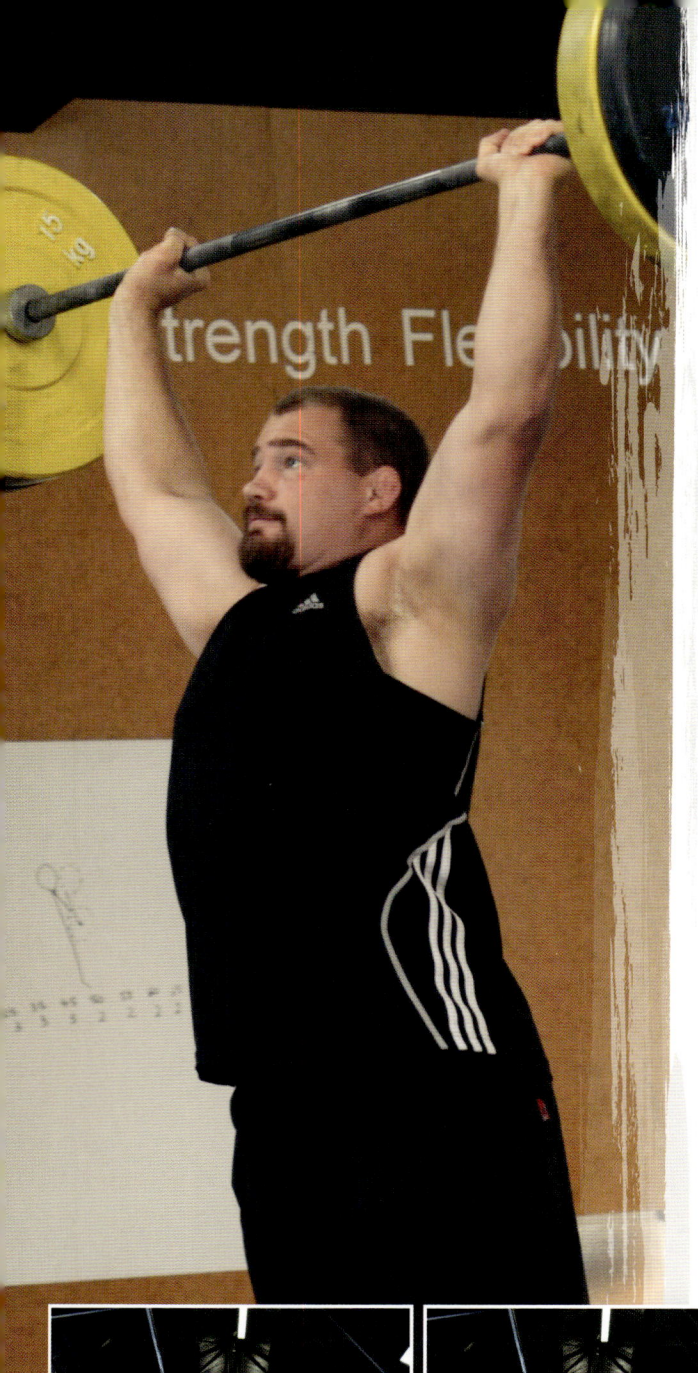

Press behind neck

Pressing behind the neck works deeper in the back of the shoulders and requires good open posture. Remember to keep your chest up high when working the bar behind the head. The movement is pretty simple and so too are the results. Controlling the weight up and down behind the head will build up some quality strength in the shoulders.

BEGINNER: Find a weight that you can lift no more than 15 reps, 3 sets.

INTERMEDIATE: Lift a heavier weight that you can repeat only 10 reps, 4 sets.

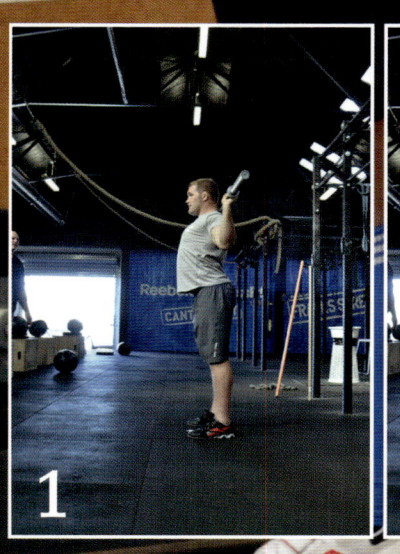

1

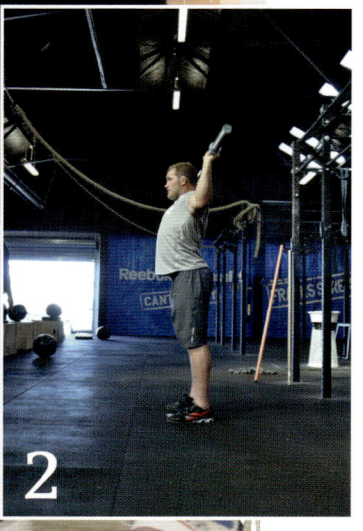

2

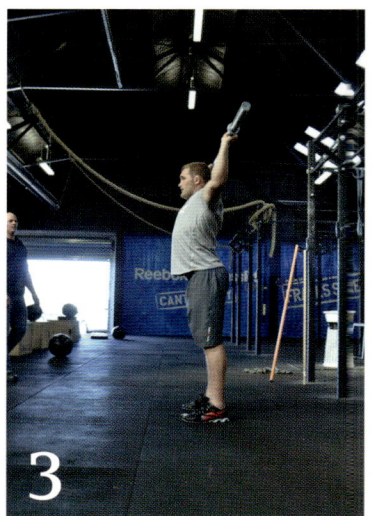

3

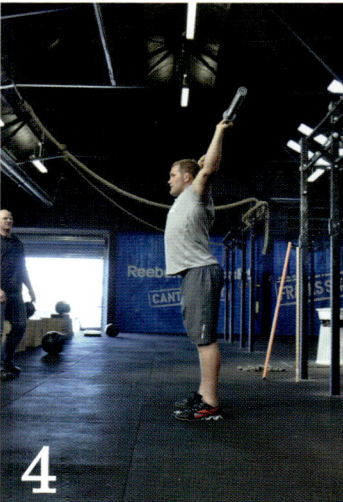

4

Push press

Designed to strengthen the top and the back of shoulder muscles, the push press is a much slower movement than the jerk or split jerk. Owen is demonstrating with a bar, but this exercise can also be done with dumbbells or if there is nothing else available, two cans of baked-beans will do. Anything that adds some resistance to get the muscles moving.

Start from a racked position, pushing the weight in a straight line up. A lot of practice will be needed for moving your head and chin out of the way of the bar when it travels in the vertical direction. Once the bar is clear of your chin, bring your head forward as far as you can to help lock the bar into position and hold for a moment. Then bring the bar back to the racked position, and repeat.

BEGINNER: Find a weight that you can lift no more than 15 reps, 3 sets.

INTERMEDIATE: Lift a heavier weight that you can repeat only 10 reps, 4 sets.

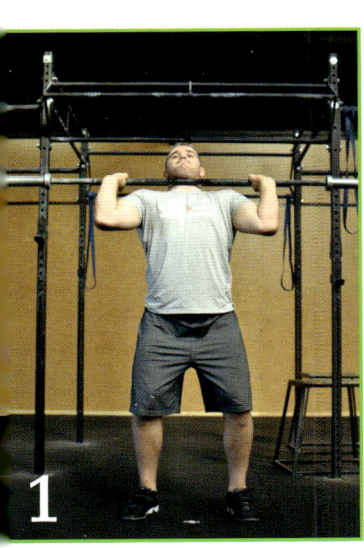
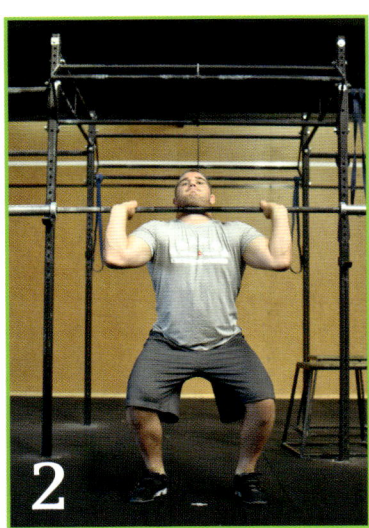
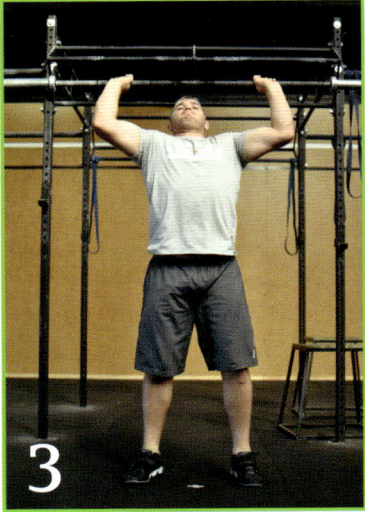
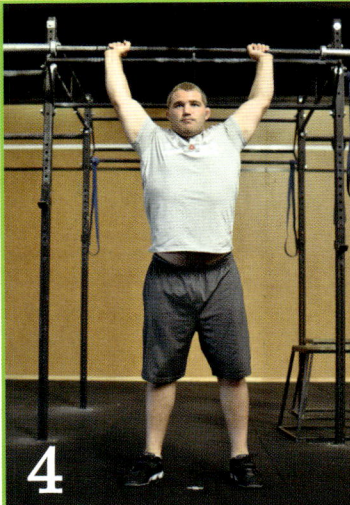

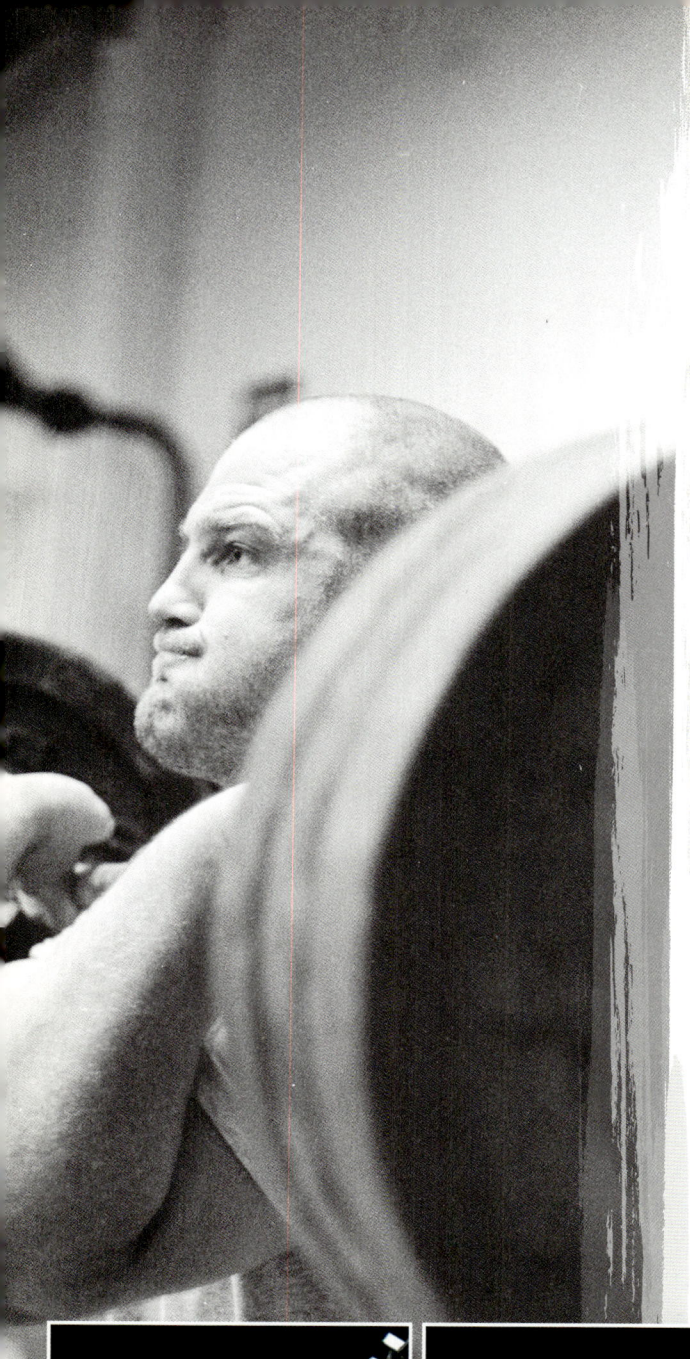

Clean and jerk

The clean and jerk is the bread and butter of powerlifting. There are two phases. The first is 'cleaning' the weight from the floor up to a racked position across the front of the shoulders. The second is the 'jerk' movement where you quickly dive under the weight, finishing with the arms outstretched.

The clean and jerk (or split jerk) is an advanced weightlifting movement. Beginners should begin with an unweighted bar or a light weight for the clean phase, and then 'push press' (see page 125) the weight for the second phase. This will be a better introduction and alternative to the explosive jerk movement.

BEGINNER: Find a weight that you can lift no more than 15 reps, 3 sets.

INTERMEDIATE: Lift a heavier weight that you can repeat only 10 reps, 4 sets.

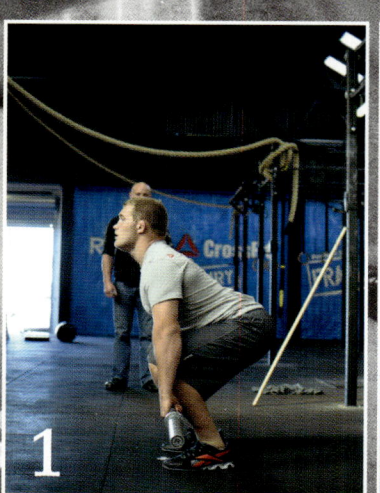
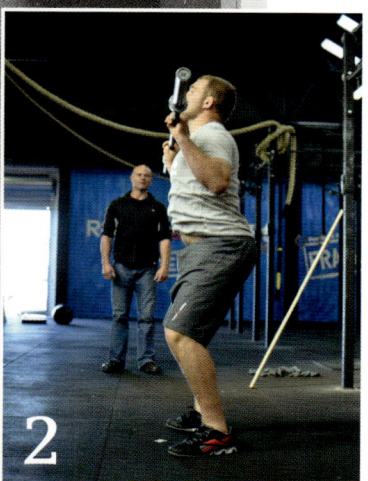
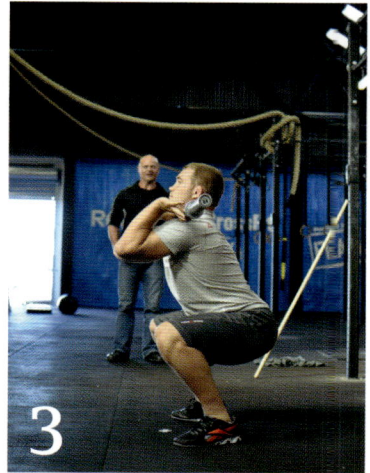
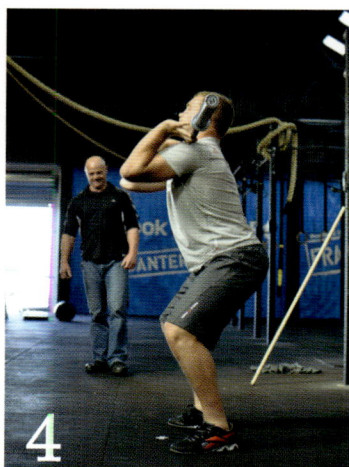

Jerk

The jerk starts with a dip to then bounce the weight slightly up, allowing enough time to slide the feet out and dive under the weight, getting quickly into position. Many hours of practice are needed to make this look as easy as Owen executing 5 sets of 3 repetitions.

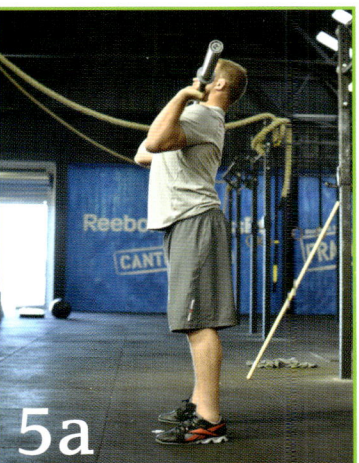 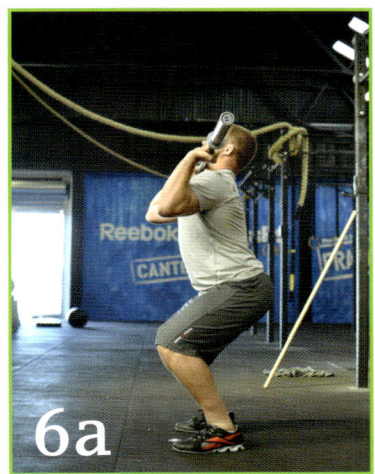 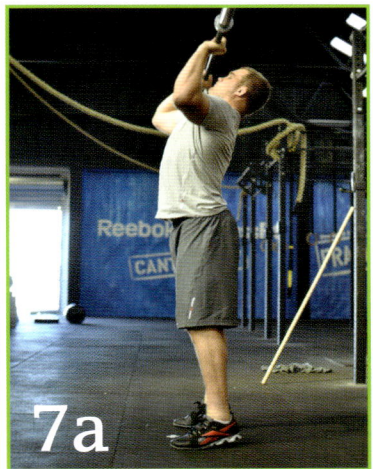 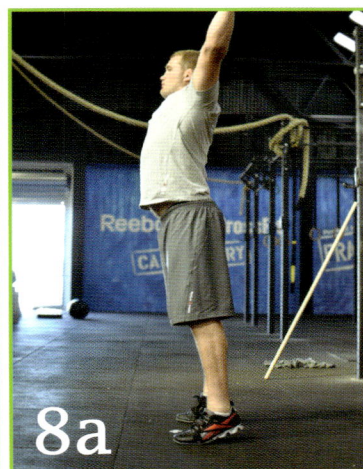

Split jerk

After a successful clean, the split jerk involves the same small bounce at the start of the jerk movement. However, when pulling yourself under the weight, only one leg bends. The other leg quickly stomps straight out behind the body with both arms locked out, balancing the weight in a central position above the head. Once stable, stand up and bring the legs together. Then safely lower the weight.

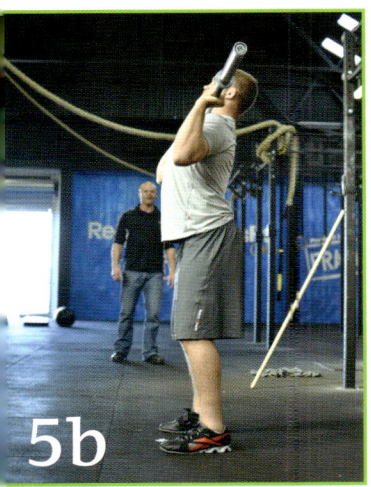 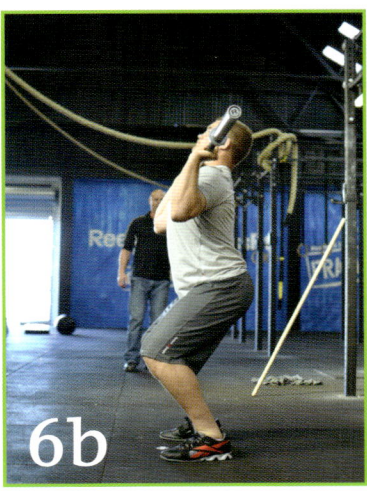 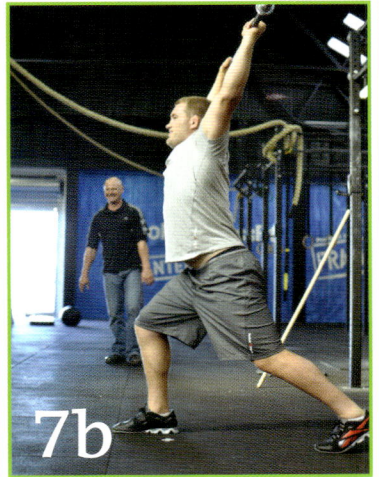 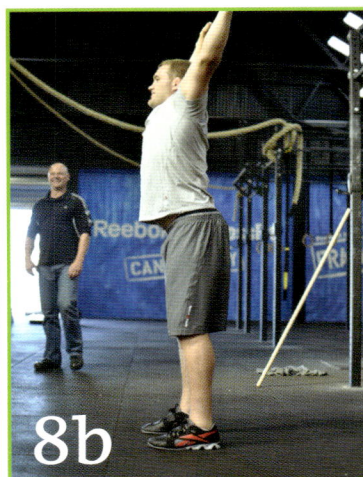

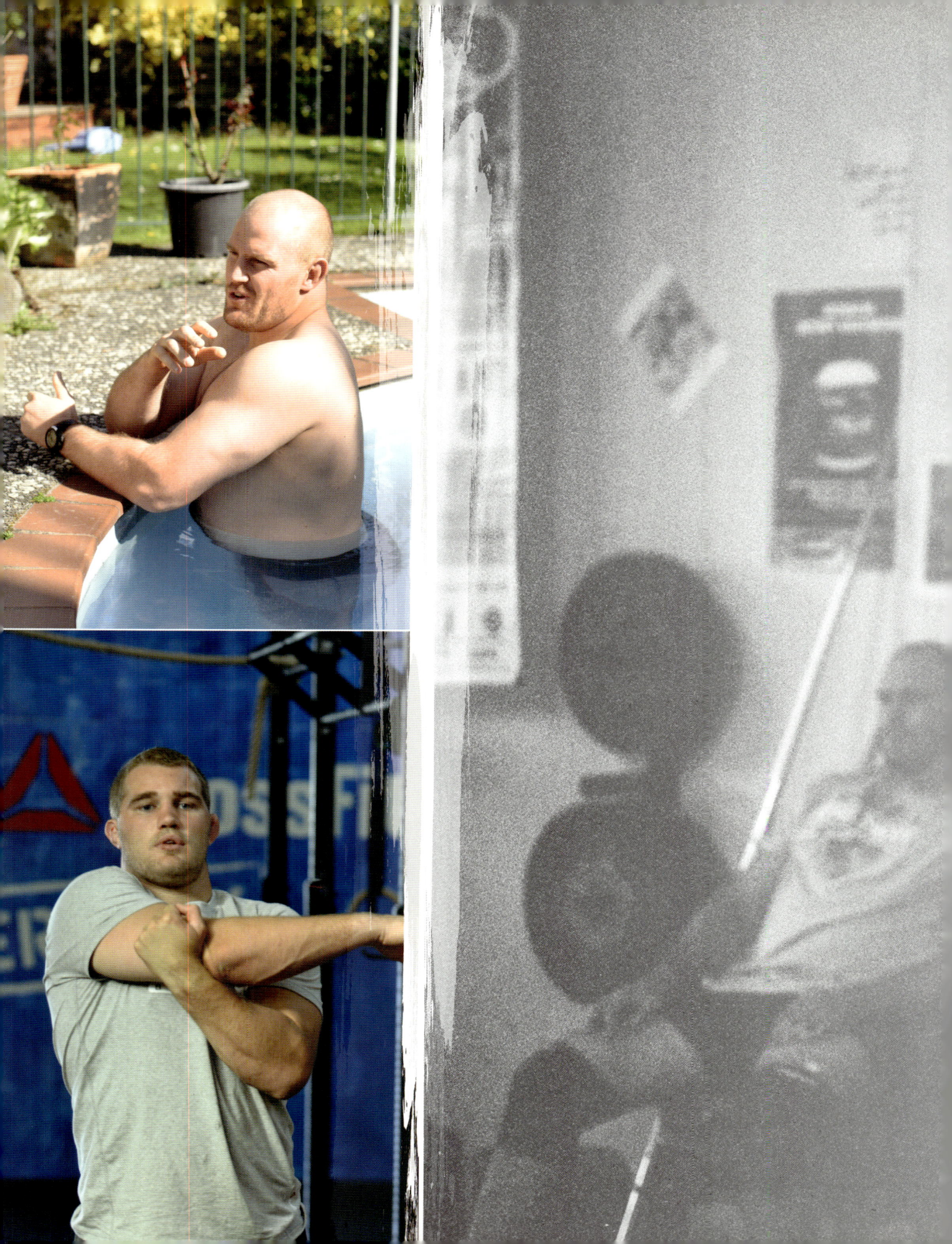

RECOVERY

Lifting weights, running hills, and training hard is actually less than half the job done. Recovery is just as, if not more, important than the exercising itself. Rehydrating, stretching, eating quality recovery foods all play a major factor in developing better performance.

Straight after training (or a game, match, bout, etc) be sure to have a drink bottle close to you so you can rehydrate, and clear out some of the lactic acid building up in your muscles. At the end of a training session both Ben and Owen also have a protein shake prepared and waiting for them. Next on the list is stretching.

Top athletes stretch. There is no better opportunity to improve your flexibility and invest in your body's longevity than straight after exercising. A light stretch is definitely recommended before exercise, but the body's temperature straight after a high-intensity workout is primed to extend your range of motion.

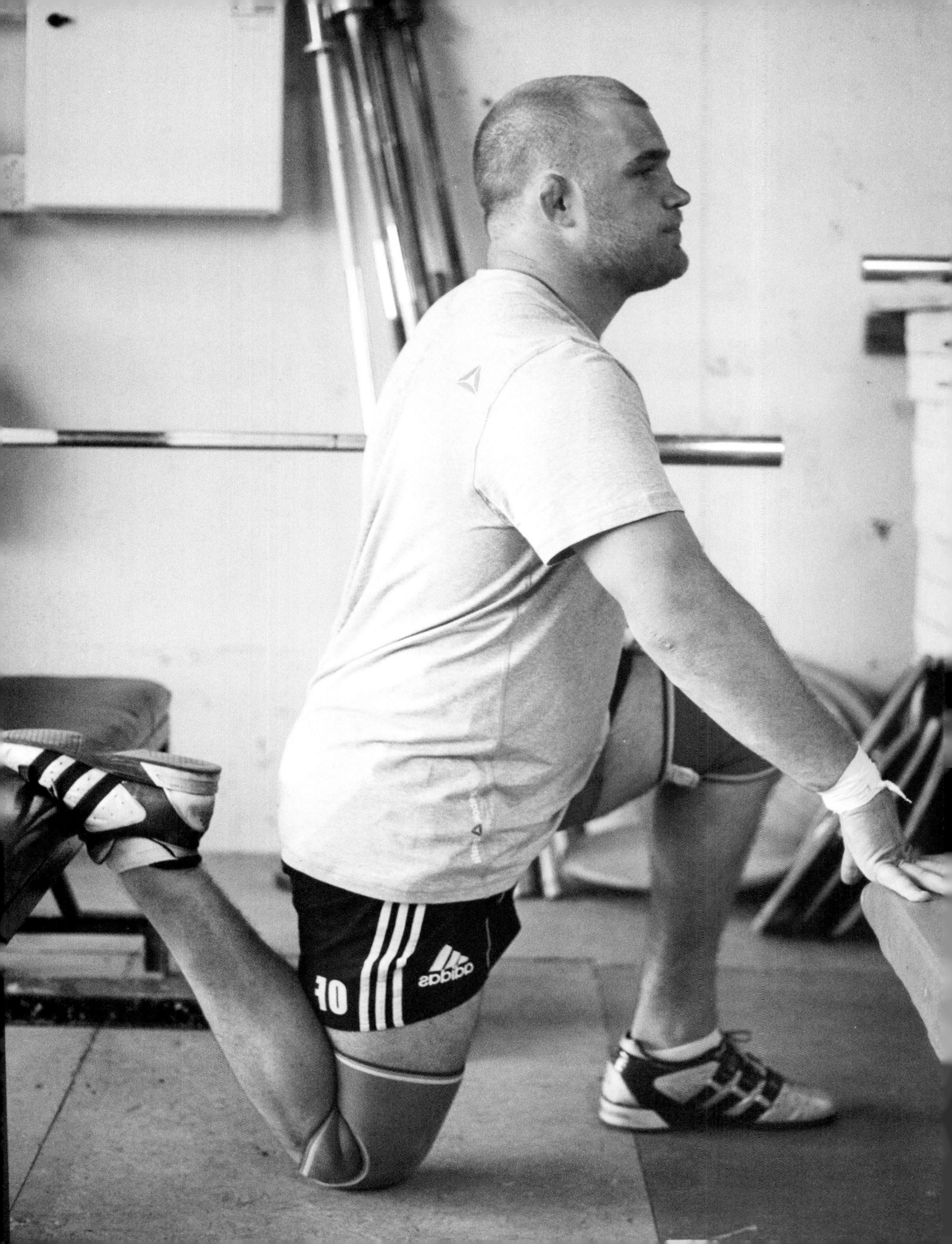

Take some time after training to sit down and stretch out, paying special attention to your major muscle groups like your back, quads and hamstring muscles in your legs. This is the time to hold and stretch the muscles for 30 seconds or longer. Slowly taking your body back through its range of motion to assure the tendons and muscles remain long and relaxed allows the muscle to grow and recover as fast as possible.

After you have cooled down it is recommended to eat some food, even if only a small amount at first. Natural food is ideal. Your body will appreciate the nutrients.

Food and diet is a huge topic, one that is well worth further researching, but to begin with some basic rules include limiting the amount of junk food you eat. A steak, potatoes, and a green salad will provide a good fix of carbohydrates and protein needed to repair used muscles and make them stronger. If you eat a 'Big Fat Combo' at the drive-through recovery time will be so much slower. Not enough quality substance comes from commercial fast-food dinners. When the Franks eat out, it's generally chicken and salad at Nando's.

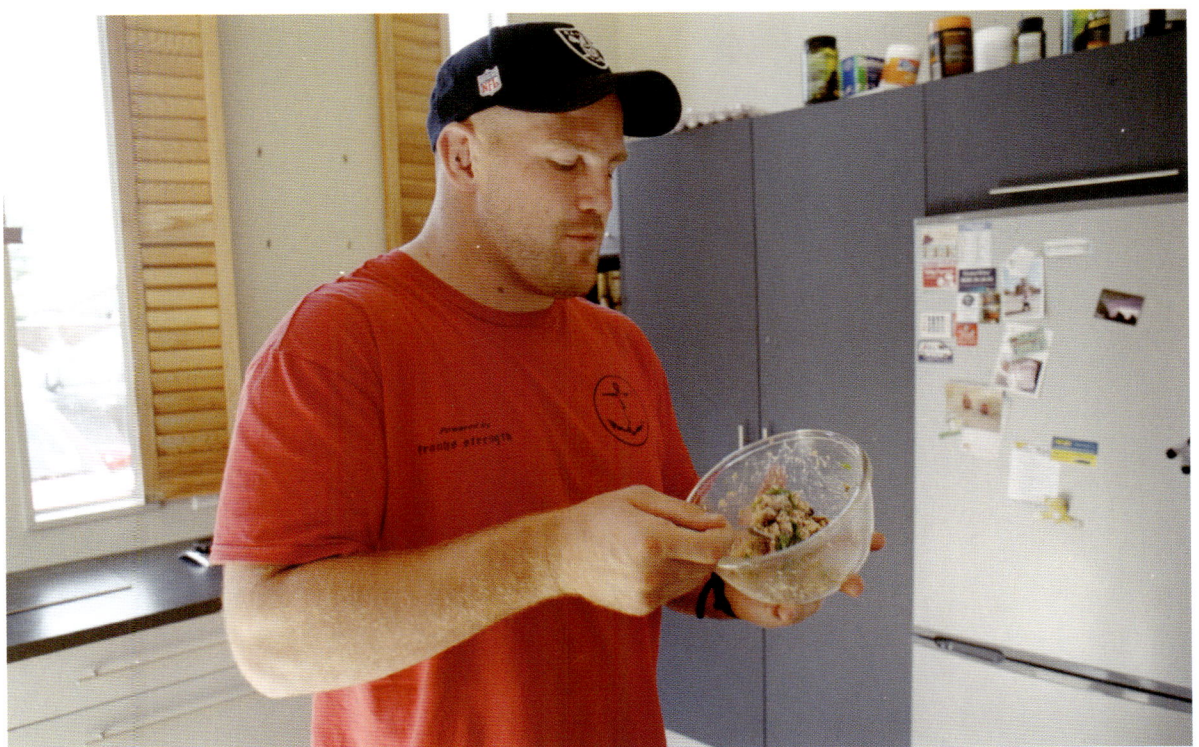

Above: Ben eating at home, making tuna salad in his kitchen in Christchurch.
Left: Ower stretching the powerful quadriceps muscle group after a heavy lifting session at Eastside Barbell, Christchurch.

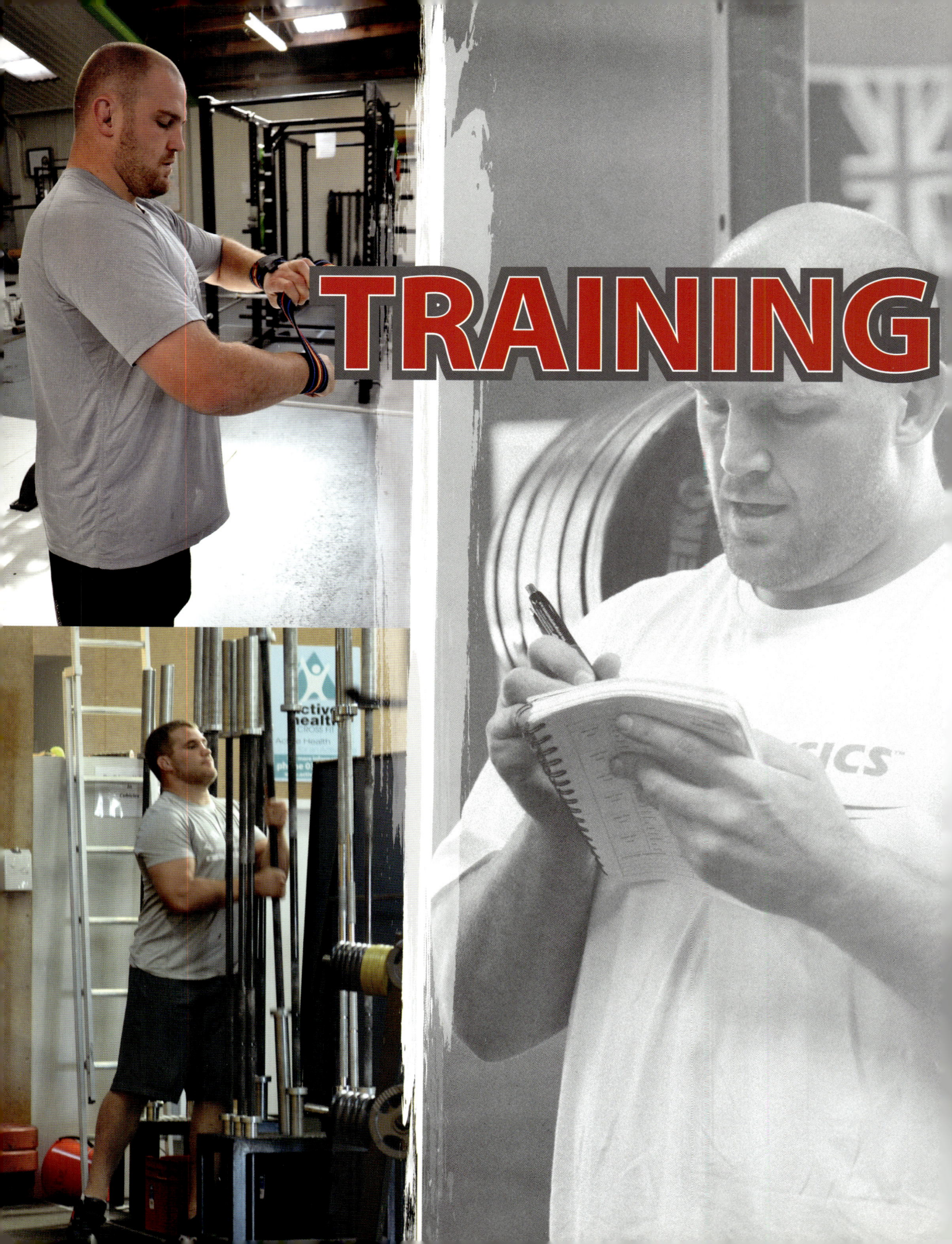

TRAINING

PROGRAM

Every effort you make to train is going to make you better. Strive to develop all aspects of fitness together, with no more emphasis placed on one particular component of fitness.

However, in order to build a sustainable training program you must first develop a large base of physical fitness. During a professional season this is called the GPP or 'General Preparation Phase' of training.

Bodyweight circuits are a wonderful way to develop the body's work capacity. Work capacity is the ability to tolerate a workload and recover from that workload. The following circuits are performed during the GPP of training. During this phase of the workout the preferred method is continuous. With developing athletes most of the training is focused on general work. Later in the athlete's training regime the general work (GPP) becomes less of a focus because training is cumulative and there is a need for more specific and technical work. (Strength and Conditioning Coach Ed Cosner)

As with all physical training a proper warm-up and cool-down is important. The great US weightlifter Tommy Kono said it best: 'If you don't have time to warm up then you don't have time to train.'

Bodyweight

Week 1	2 circuits with 30 seconds between exercises and 2 minutes between circuits.
Weeks 2 & 3	2 circuits with 15 seconds between exercises and 1 minute between circuits.
Week 4	3 circuits with 15 seconds between exercises and 1 minute between circuits.
Weeks 5 & 6	3 circuits with no rest between exercises and no rest between circuits.

Circuit: Day 1

Requires some open floor space, a solid box or chair to step up, and a pull-up bar.

EXERCISE	REPS/DISTANCE	NOTE	PAGE
1. Air squats	x 20	Place hands behind your head to ensure an upright body position.	73
2. Push-ups	x 10	To help keep good form, don't allow your hips to touch the floor throughout all 10 reps.	75
3. Alternate leg step-ups	x 10 (each leg)	The box or bench should be tall enough so that when the leg is on the bench the thigh is parallel to the ground.	76
4. Pull-ups (underhand)	x 8	Use a narrow underhand grip. Pointing your toes makes it easier.	77
5. Alternate lunges	x 10 (each leg)	Either alternating the step forward (back leg almost touching the ground), then stepping back to the same position, or if you have room in front of you stepping forward.	78
6. Pull-ups (overhand)	x 8	Use an overhand grip. Pointing your toes makes it easier.	77
7. Air squats	x 20	Place hands behind your head to ensure an upright body position.	73

8. Bear crawl	20 m	Try to stay on your hands and feet for the full 2 minutes. Otherwise have a 30 second break between each minute to build up more strength.	80
9. Sit-ups	x 20	If you are really keen, do as many as you can to finish Day 1's circuit.	69

Circuit: Day 2

Ideally requires a hill or slope to add resistance.

EXERCISE	REPS/DISTANCE	NOTE	PAGE
1. Bear crawl	20 m	10 metres forward and 10 metres backward. Run on your hands and feet as fast as you can forwards and back 10 metres.	80
2. Hill sprint	20 m	Run at your 100 per cent max speed and catch your breath before beginning bear crawls.	82
3. Bear crawl	20 m	Bear crawl x 10 metres right and x 10 metres left. Move your hands and feet sideways as fast as you can.	80
4. Lateral slides	10 m	Swap leading legs on each circuit repetition.	82
5. Hill sprint	20 m	Run at your 100 per cent max speed and catch your breath before beginning bear crawls.	82

Basic strength training

This is a very basic training program designed to begin to develop strength, which is the basis of all movement.

EXERCISE	BEGINNER		INTERMEDIATE		PAGE
	REPS	SETS	REPS	SETS	
MONDAY					
1. Bench press	15	3	10	4	37
2. Seated shoulder press	15	3	10	4	38
3. Lat pull-downs	15	3	10	4	39
4. Triceps extensions	15	3	10	4	91
5. Barbell curls	15	3	10	4	93
TUESDAY					
1. Front squats	15	3	10	4	95
2. Dead lifts	15	3	10	4	97
3. Dumbbell rows	15	3	10	4	99
4. Sit-ups	15	3	10	4	59
FRIDAY					
1. Back squats	15	3	10	4	103
2. Cleans from floor	15	3	10	4	120–121
3. Toes to bar	15	3	10	4	71
4. Calf raiser	15	3	10	4	104

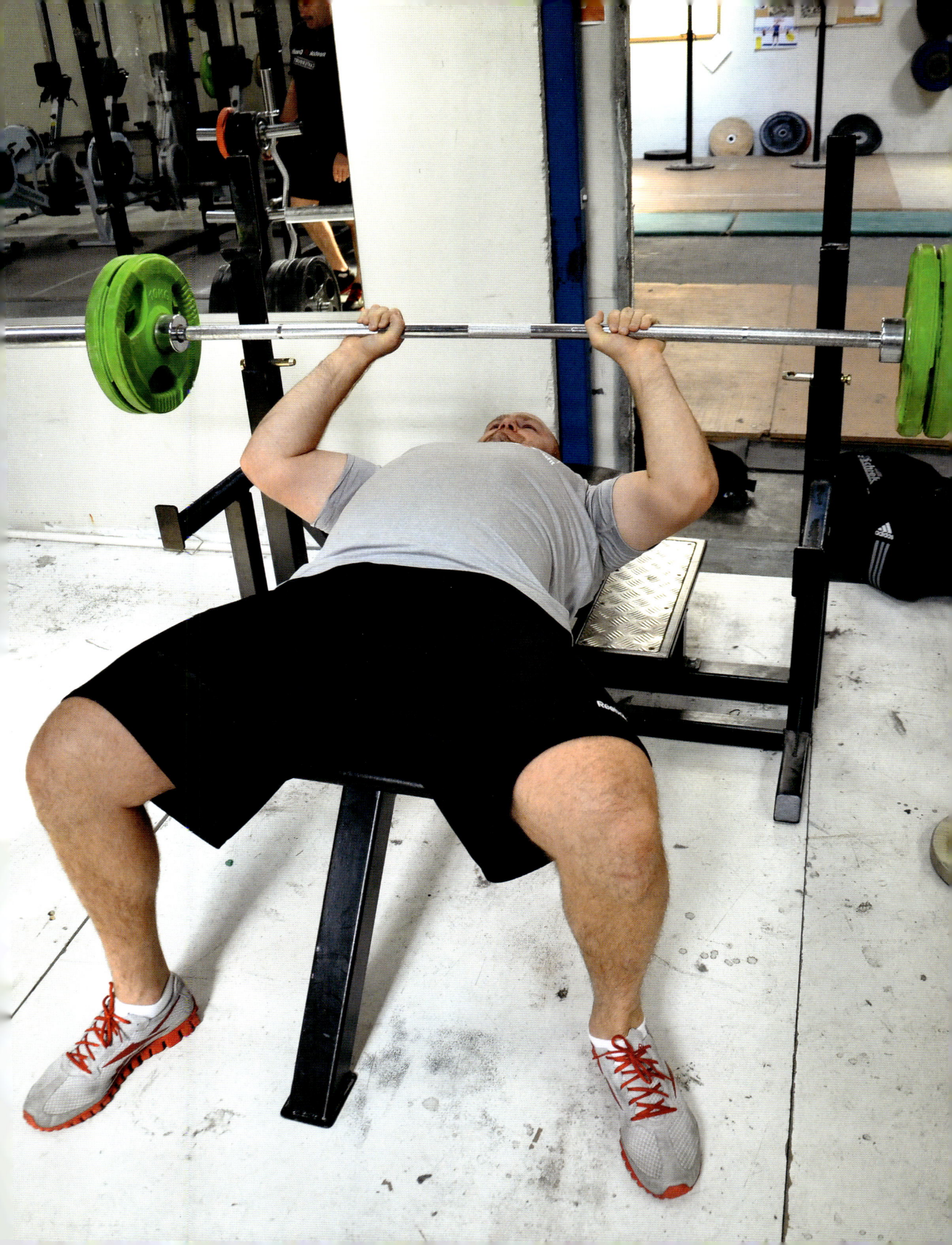

Olympic Weightlifting Power Program

EXERCISE	REPS	SETS	PAGE
DAY 1			
1. Snatch squat	x3	5	108
2. Drop snatch	x3	5	109
3. Snatch from waist	x3	5	110
4. Snatch from hang	x3	5	111
5. Snatch pull	x3	5	112
6. Front squat	x3	4	95
8. Core exercises (Alternate between sit-ups, leg raisers, and toes to bar)	x10	5	68–83
DAY 2			
1. Front squat	x3	4	95
2. Clean from waist	x3	5	117
3. Clean from hang	x3	5	118
4. Clean from floor	x3	5	121
5. Clean pull	x3	5	122
8. Core exercises (Alternate between sit-ups, leg raisers, and toes to bar)	x10	5	68–83

EXERCISE	REPS	SETS	PAGE
DAY 3			
1. Snatch/Power snatch from floor	x3	5	113
2. Clean & jerk or push press	x2	5	125, 126
3. Back squat	x3	5	103
4. Clean pull	x3	5	122
FINISHER: Just to make sure every muscle group is fully spent, finish the training week with the following 6 exercises:			
1. Upright row	x10 to 20	3	100
2. Triceps extension	x10 to 20	3	91
3. Press behind neck	x10 to 20	3	124
4. Bicep curls with bar or dumbells	x10 to 20	3	93
5. Push-ups	x10 to 20	3	75
6. Leg raisers	x10 to 20	3	70

Ken's CrossFit

STRENGTH & CONDITIONING
Work out of the Day

If you race for your best time over the full 5 rounds of this workout, it will not only challenge your muscles but also give your heart and lungs a really good workout — improving your overall fitness.

EXERCISE	REPS	SETS	NOTE	PAGE
1. Cleans from hang	x12	5	To find the right weight, build up slowly starting with just the weight of the bar. Slowly increase until you find a weight that you CANNOT lift more than 6 continuous reps. When attempting each round of Hang Cleans you need at least one rest in the middle (6 x 6 or in the last few rounds (4 x 4 x 4). However you break the set up, you must complete 12 before moving onto Triceps Dip.	118
2. Triceps dip	x12	5	Using your arm's full range of motion, lower your body keeping your hips forward — don't allow them to sag. If you find your own body weight too light, place a 10 or 20 kg plate on your lap.	81
EXTRA				
If after your workout you feel you want to do more, allow some time to recover then do the following				
3. 200 m sprints	x1	4–8	Time each sprint and rest 1 minute between sets.	n/a

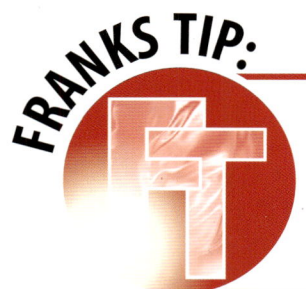

FRANKS TIP:

Try to keep your sprint times within 5 seconds of each other.